Nicholas Bjorn

particularly good for snacking on and you will find that many restaurants provide them as an alternative to bread.

Egg Whites

The egg debate is an age-old one. Some people say the yolks are fine to eat, others say they are not okay to eat and that you should only eat egg whites. Whole eggs are a fantastic source of protein and the biggest debate rages around the cholesterol and fat levels in the yolks. If you want to be safe, eat the whites on and start adding yolks back in at a later date.

Grapefruit

Grapefruits are an excellent fat burning food and this is being proved with more research every year. Grapefruit helps to kick start the digestive system, making fat burning an easier and more efficient process. You can start with pure grapefruit juice if you want and work your way up to eating a grapefruit.

Chicken Breast

Chicken breast is a staple part of many diets, although it is obviously no good if you are going vegetarian or vegan. It is low in fat and high in protein and is far healthier to eat than the dark meat from a chicken. Do remember to take the skin off, as this is where all the fat is and use a variety of spices and herbs to boost the flavor. Combine eating chicken breast with strength training to help tone up your muscles, which will boost your metabolism rate as well.

Wheat Grass

Wheatgrass is a superfood made out of the Triticum Aestivum plant. It contains high amounts of nutrients that are great for your health. It is generally consumed in the form of fresh juice, but nowadays, it is also available in the form of powder. The powder is far more convenient than the juice. While a lot of people now understand the importance of wheatgrass, many people are still unaware of its benefits, which is why it still remains an underrated superfood. If consumed daily, wheatgrass can help you tackle many diseases and disorders.

As said above, wheatgrass is full of a variety of nutrients that are necessary for our body. Wheatgrass also has many nourishing and therapeutic properties. It contains many different vitamins and minerals that keep fit and active. It also contains a variety of enzymes that are good for your digestive system. Another factor that makes wheatgrass really great is that it improves and enhances the immune system. It is also good for people who are trying to lose weight because it tackles cholesterol levels and minimizes them. Wheatgrass also makes you calm and relaxed. It can relieve you of anxiety. It improves mental function. It reduces stress. It improves cognitive function and can also be used to prevent the symptoms of Alzheimer's disease.

Salmon

Salmon is a highly nutritious fish that is considered to be an important superfood. It contains high amounts of omega three and healthy fats. The nutrients and oil present in salmon are rarely found in other species of fish, which makes salmon one of the healthiest fish. Salmon contains a high amount of polyunsaturated fats. These fats reduce the levels of serum triglycerides and can enhance brain functioning and cardiovascular health as well.

It is true that salmon is a pricey seafood option, but the number of nutrients (and taste) present in it makes it worth it. It metabolism and thus can lead to efficient fat burning. It has other antioxidants that can help you prevent cancer.

There are various bioactive compounds present in green tea, which are good for the health of your brain. They can reduce the effects of Parkinson's and Alzheimer's effectively. These two are the most common neurodegenerative disorders. Green tea contains a high amount of catechins, which can reduce the growth of certain viruses and bacteria. This is turn can reduce infections and can also improve your oral and dental health. It is also effective against halitosis.

In certain controlled trials, it was observed that green tea could also reduce blood sugar levels and thus can reduce the risk of Type 2 diabetes as well. Green tea can also reduce LDL cholesterol. Thus, green tea can help you live longer and look young for a long time as well.

Apples

Apples are one of the best fruits, as they contain no cholesterol or fats. They also contain no sodium and are a great low-calorie snack. Apples are not only delicious, but they are also highly nutritious. Apples contain high amounts of dietary fiber. It is estimated that one medium-sized fruit contains around 5 grams of dietary fiber. Apples are a rich source of soluble fiber, which is good for satiation. This is why apples are often an integral part of the diet of people who are trying to lose weight. Apples keep you feeling full for a long time.

Apples contain high amounts of vitamin C along with fiber. They are also a rich source of polyphenols. Polyphenols have multiple health benefits and are great for your cardiovascular health. Apples also contain nutrients that can help you to lower your cholesterol levels. According to studies, eating apples regularly can also help you lower the risk of Type 2 diabetes.

itself. Start to push yourself harder and harder – if you get comfortable doing your training, your weight loss will simply plateau. If you are not breaking a sweat through your exercise, you are not working out hard enough. If you are not sweating, you are not burning fat and your heart rate is not working to your benefit.

If you are looking to burn fat, you need to create an extreme energy demand so that your body is able to change. Lifting the same old weights time and time again will not help you to burn fat and you won't be gaining any real benefits from your physical activity.

Mistake Number 6 – You are doing too much low intensity cardio training

Ok, so I just told you to up the intensity of your workout and now I'm telling you off for doing too much of something that isn't intensive. Cardio is not a form of resistance training. It is a completely different type of fitness and a two-hour slog on the treadmill is not going to give you the results that an hour of heavy lifting will.

If you want your cardio to work, do full body workouts that include a short rest period. By using your whole body and taking shorter breaks, your cardiovascular system and your muscular system are being challenged.

Mistake Number 7 – You are stressed out

Stress is one of the biggest and most silent killers. Stress causes your body to produce cortisol in levels way beyond what is normal. This can be responsible to an increase in fat storage in the body and many other negative consequences. Even if your diet and your training regime are spot-on, if you re stressed, you will not achieve your goals.

Nicholas Bjorn

sitting. Now, when you eat a calorie deficit and then strength train, your body gets even cleverer and stronger over time, resulting in serious weight loss without any loss in muscle mass.

Now, here's a scenario for you: You are weight training, your muscles are breaking down and need rebuilding. Because you are eating less than usual, there aren't enough calories ingested as compared to the number needed for the rebuilding process. So, what happens? Is it not worth doing all of this?

Of course not!

This is where our amazing body comes into play. Remember the "Reserve Store of Fats"? Yep. The body pulls out calories from this reserve stock and happily goes about rebuilding the muscles. You just need to keep eating enough and eat foods based on your exercise and diet goals.

Resting properly is also an important part of rebuilding muscle and keeping them strong for the next workout. This, in turn, will promote hunger at the right time, and you will eat only the right foods for your body.

CHIA Green Smoothie

- 1 scoop whey protein vanilla
- 1 tbsp. chia seeds
- 1 cup spinach
- 1 cup almond milk
- 1 banana
- water/ice

The Winter Mint Chocolate Shake

- 1 scoop whey protein , chocolate or chocolate mint
- 1 cup almond milk
- 1/2 cup arctic zero mint chocolate
- 1 drop peppermint extract
- 2 ice cubes

Green Spinach-Apple-Mango Yogurt Smoothie

- 3/4 cup plain 0% Greek yogurt
- 1/2 bunch spinach
- 1 apple
- 1/2 cup mango chunks
- 1 cup ice/water

Stop Dieting & Weight Loss Motivation

How To Stop Dieting And Eat Normally

& The Ultimate MotivationGuide

By Nicholas Bjorn

Nicholas Bjorn

Book 1
Stop Dieting

How to Stop Dieting and Eat Normally

The Best Healthy Weight Loss Foods to Eat

3rd Edition

By Nicholas Bjorn

Nicholas Bjorn

© Copyright 2021 – All rights reserved.

The contents of this book may not be reproduced, duplicated, or transmitted without direct written permission from the author.

Under no circumstances will any legal responsibility or blame be held against the publisher for any reparation, damages, or monetary loss due to the information herein, either directly or indirectly.

Legal Notice:

This book is copyright protected. This is only for personal use. You cannot amend, distribute, sell, use, quote, or paraphrase any part of the content within this book without the consent of the author.

Disclaimer Notice:

Please note the information contained within this document is for educational and entertainment purposes only. Every attempt has been made to provide accurate, up-to-date, complete, and reliable information. No warranties of any kind are expressed or implied. Readers acknowledge that the author is not engaging in the rendering of legal, financial, medical, or professional advice. The content of this book has been derived from various sources. Please consult a licensed professional before attempting any techniques outlined in this book.

By reading this document, the reader agrees that under no circumstances is the author responsible for any losses, direct or indirect, which are incurred as a result of the use of information contained within this document, including, but not limited to, errors, omissions, or inaccuracies.

Nicholas Bjorn

Table of Contents

Introduction 11

Chapter 1 – 10 Nutrition Rules for Boosting Energy Burning Fat 15

Chapter 2 – Top 10 Herbs and Spices to Help Improve Health and Weight Loss 21

Chapter 3 – 36 Fat Burning Super Foods 25

Chapter 4 - The Top 20 Superfoods You Should be Eating 37

Chapter 5 – 8 Reasons Why You Are Not Losing Body Fat 67

Chapter 6 – Eat Right For Weight Loss 73
   Basal Metabolic Rate (BMR) 74
   Metabolism and Weight Loss 76
   What Else Can I Do? 80

Chapter 7 – Planning Your Meals 85

Chapter 8 – The Importance of Water 89
   Benefits of Drinking Water 89
   How Much Water Should I Drink? 93
   Water and its Many Forms 94
   The Role of Water in Weight Loss 94

Chapter 9 – Strength Training: A Vital Component of Your Weight Loss Journey 97

Chapter 10 – Kitchen Implements and Gadgets for Healthy Cooking 99

Chapter 11 – Refrigerator Essentials for Healthy Eating 103
For Your Freezer 105

Chapter 12 – How to Eat Healthy Without Going Broke and Losing Your Mind 107
Shopping the Right Way for Health 107

Chapter 13 – 15 Tasty Super Food Smoothies Recipes 111
Peanut Butter Power Shake 111
Dark Chocolate Shake 111
CHIA Green Smoothie 112
The Winter Mint Chocolate Shake 112
Green Spinach-Apple-Mango Yogurt Smoothie 112
Anti-Aging Kiwi-Blueberry Smoothie 113
Berry Banana Smoothie 113
Peach-Mango Yogurt Smoothie 114
The Lean Muscle Mochaccino 114
Orange Creamsicle Smoothie 114
Liquid Breakfast Smoothie 115
Banana Nut Shake 115
Strawberry Shortcake Smoothie 115
Mango Pineapple Shake 116
Creamy Chocolate Avocado Smoothie 116

Chapter 14 – 5 Tasty Super Food Soup Recipes 117
Green Superfood Soup 117
Carrot and Turmeric Soup 119

Dairy-Free Creamy Avocado Soup 121

Spicy Chicken and Quinoa Soup 122

Slow Cooker Superfood Soup 124

Chapter 15 – 6 Yummy and Healthy One-Bowl Meals 127

Quinoa and Chicken Burrito Bowl with Green Sauce 127

French Lentil Salad with Goat Cheese 131

Thai Chicken Soup with Rice Noodles 133

Cauliflower Fried Rice 135

Thai Shrimp and Quinoa 137

Ratatouille Rice 139

Chapter 16 – Sweet Endings: Lip Smacking Healthy Desserts 141

Avocado Chocolate Mousse with Summer Fruit 141

Raspberry Vegan Cheesecake 143

Cinnamon Baked Pears 145

Healthy Peanut Butter Fudge 146

No-Bake Brownie Energy Bites 148

Apple Crumble 149

Yogurt Cocktail 151

Quick Coffee Dessert 153

Simple Rice Pudding 155

Rich Chocolate Slices 156

Conclusion 159

References 163

Nicholas Bjorn

Introduction

This book includes proven steps and strategies on how you can boost energy and burn fat, plus the best fat burning super foods you should be eating for healthy weight loss.

If you have tried to lose weight before, you know it's not always easy. With so many diets to choose from and each telling you're a different way to eat and what foods to avoid; it can easily get confusing or frustrating. That's why this book focuses on normal foods you can actually eat to not only lose weight, but also improve your health.

If you are truly serious about losing weight and are prepared to make the commitment to eating healthier, then this is the book for you.

Nicholas Bjorn

Stop Dieting

FREE E-BOOKS SENT WEEKLY

Join North Star Readers Book Club
And Get Exclusive Access To The Latest Kindle Books in
Health, Fitness, Weight Loss and Much More...

TO GET YOU STARTED HERE IS YOUR FREE E-BOOK:

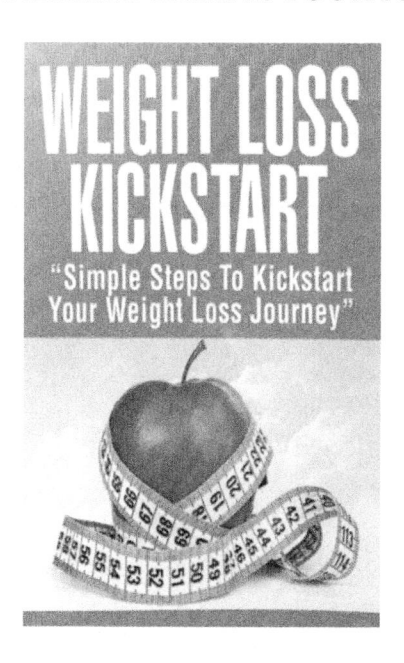

Visit to Sign Up Today!
www.northstarreaders.com/weight-loss-kick-start

Chapter 1 – 10 Nutrition Rules for Boosting Energy Burning Fat

Everyone wants to feel good, to feel alert, rested and full of energy but, for most, this is just a dream. The reality is we live in a harsh world, where time is in short supply and stress is in abundance. Lack of sleep combined with poor diet and stress leads to illness and exhaustion.

Fatigue is one of the worst things for the human body; it breaks us down emotionally and physically and it wreaks total havoc on our immune systems, which opens the way for chronic disease. But we all have the power needed to make that change, to give our bodies the energy boost they need and to feel fantastic with it.

Regular exercise, learning how to manage stress and sleeping properly are all critical factors in being able to combat fatigue but you can also make a change to your eating habits. The following are ten ways in which you can use the food you eat to give you energy that lasts throughout the day.

Rule Number 1 – Eat Foods that are Dense in Nutrients

The best way to boost your metabolism to convert your food into energy is eat foods that contain the right minerals and vitamins – and plenty of them. If you eat the right food, all the cells in your body will produce energy to keep you going.

Rule Number 2 – Eat Foods that are High in Antioxidants

These are the scavengers that clean out all the chemicals and toxins in the body that are wearing you down. Eat plenty of fruits and vegetables and other plant-based foods rather than taking them in supplement form. Eating too much of some nutrients can be risky so get round this by eating only whole foods, like colorful berries, melons and dark green leafy vegetables.

Rule Number 3 – Eating your Omega-3's

Over the years, research has shown that plenty of omega-3 in your diet can improve your memory, mood and thinking, all of which are closely related to energy. Try to eat one good helping per day in the form of flax oil or seeds, fish, hemp oil or seeds, leafy greens and walnuts.

Rule Number 4 – Stop Dieting

Most diets are no good for the human body because they require you to deprive your body of certain foods. You should not cut your calories down too much because this just decreases your metabolism. That is why many people who are on strict diets often complain of lethargy. And, as your metabolism slows down, your body will burn off less calories, which means the ultimate result, is a gain in weight. Eat the right amount of calorie needs every day and eat them in the right foods, combined with regular exercise if you want to successfully drop the pounds.

Rule Number 5 – Don't Skip Breakfast

Yes, it is so easy, when you are running late and there are those who think that to lose weight they have to skip a meal. It is the wrong meal to skip. Breakfast is the most important meal of the day as it gets your metabolism off and running and a good breakfast will keep your energy levels up until it's time for lunch. Instead of hitting the bagel bar or eating stodgy cereals, go for eggs, fresh fruit, whole grain cereal and nuts.

Rule Number 6 – Don't Pass on Snacks

It is important to eat enough of the right foods to keep you blood glucose levels steady throughout the day, and that will keep your energy levels steady as well. Snack on dried fruit and nuts, yoghurt with granola, whole grain crackers, fresh raw vegetables and fruits.

Rule Number 7 – Drink Your Fluids

Hydration is an important part of weight loss and of keeping your energy levels high. Your body needs a lot of water to function at its best but, unless you are doing endurance training, skip the energy drinks and vitamin waters. Instead, drink plain water or water with fresh fruit chunks in it and aim to drink at least one cup every couple of hours.

Rule Number 8 – Be a Designated Driver

That will help you to cut out one of the biggest enemies of those who want to lose weight – alcohol. As well as acting as a depressant, alcohol can also act as a stimulant, interrupting your sleep patterns and causing tiredness the following day. If you are relying on a drink every night to help you fall asleep, you are doing the wrong thing. Cutting out the alcohol will help you to sleep better.

If you do want to have a drink occasionally, stick to red wine. It is an antioxidant but do be aware that you cannot drink if you are on certain medications, have high blood pressure or anxiety.

Rule Number 9 – Caffeine – Little or None

Caffeine should be used carefully and in small amounts. Although it seems as if it is giving you an energy boost, it won't last for long and you will know it when it wears off. And never use caffeine as a meal replacement! Green tea is a better choice of caffeine as it also contains antioxidants and theanine, which is an essential amino acid that helps you to stay calm.

Rule Number 10 – Eat Power Foods

Try to stick to nutritional foods that provide energy, a list of 10 are below. Later on I will go into more details on foods to eat to help you burn off fat.

- Nuts, especially almonds
- Avocado
- Dark leafy greens, such as watercress, kale, spinach, collard or beet greens
- Whole grains that are intact, like quinoa, millet, brown rice or amaranth
- Ground flax seeds
- White beans, lentils, black beans
- Dried fruits such as dates but in moderation
- Berries – blackberries, strawberries, raspberries, blueberries, etc.
- Sea vegetables such as Nori, hijiki, dulse, etc.

- Edamame – whole young soy beans

Nicholas Bjorn

Chapter 2 – Top 10 Herbs and Spices to Help Improve Health and Weight Loss

Herbs and spices are a fantastic way of giving otherwise bland food a taste boost and using them is one of the best ways to enjoy nutritious foods that may not taste so great. Not many people know that herbs and spices are full of health benefits. The following are ten of the best to boost your health and excite your taste buds.

Cayenne Pepper

Adds a dash of spice and also helps to enhance bodily functions. Cayenne helps to boost the metabolism, in turn increasing the amount of fat that your body burns off and it improves your blood flow. This means that the essential nutrients and vitamins in your food are moved through the body far more efficiently, allowing your body to function better.

Black Pepper

Similar to cayenne, black pepper helps to boost the metabolism and it helps to improve the digestive process, which in turn helps the body to shed weight. It also contains anti-cancer properties.

Ginger

Ginger is good for suppressing the appetite and aiding digestion. It also works to warm up the body, increasing metabolism and helping more calories to burn off. Ginger is good for shifting toxins out of the body, in particular out of the fat cells.

Ginseng

Ginseng helps to boost metabolism and raise energy levels and is popular in energy drinks. It is a great one to use just before you do short high intensity workouts.

Chamomile Tea

Chamomile tea is great for relaxation and helps to reduce stress levels. It also helps to stop emotional eating in the evenings, thus preventing weight gain and it helps you to sleep better. Chamomile contains anti-inflammatory properties, helping to reduce the inflammation that causes so many different diseases, and it is high in antioxidants, eliminating free radicals from the body.

Cumin

Cumin tends to be mixed with other spices to give a nice flavor to Mexican, Indian, Middle Eastern and Mediterranean foods. It is used as a part of Ayurvedic medicine, helps to boost your immune system, decrease your cholesterol and contains anti-oxidant properties. It helps to increase the energy levels, allowing for more calories to be burned off.

Turmeric

Turmeric is fantastic for people who crave junk food. It helps to boost the function of the liver and to balance out hormones, which also prevents binges. It is a powerful antioxidant that helps to maintain good joints and skin, as well as vision. It works to enhance the immune system, digestive processes and the function of the liver as well as stabilizing blood glucose levels and cutting down on the amount of fat storage.

Cinnamon

This is a sweet spice that helps to boost metabolism and improve insulin sensitivity, thus helping to boost fat burning and control the blood sugar levels.

Mustard

Mustard helps to boost weight loss because it is full of B-complex vitamins, such as niacin, folates, riboflavin and thiamine, all of which increase the metabolism. One teaspoon of mustard can help to boost metabolism by 25%. Mustard is also high in magnesium and selenium which provides anti-inflammatory properties to help fight off disease. It is also a good source of zeaxanthins, carotenes and luteins, all of which are good antioxidants that help to eliminate free radicals.

Cardamom

This is a sweet spice that is used in Indian cooking and it helps to promote a healthy digestion and increases your metabolism. It is a commonly used ingredient in Ayurvedic medicine and has been shown to help mouth ulcers, high blood pressure, and depression. It has both anti-oxidative and anti-inflammatory properties and can also help to slow down the aging process.

So, the next time you are preparing your meals, add in one or more of these herbs and spices. Not only will your food taste nicer, your health will be better and your metabolism will be faster, helping you to burn off fat more efficiently.

Chapter 3 – 36 Fat Burning Super Foods

Food is not our enemy but so many diets will have you believe that it is. You don't need to eat a diet that is lacking in taste or looks to lose weight and you certainly do not need to deprive yourself just because the latest fad diet says you mustn't at certain foods. The following 36 foods are super foods that will help you to burn off fat more efficiently. However, don't get stuck on just one of them; introduce a few of them at a time to your weekly menu and, as time goes on, you will find that you are eating more and more of them.

Tomatoes

Who really cares if a tomato is a fruit or a vegetable? All that is important is knowing that a tomato contains loads of goodness that can help your body in the long terms and, over the short term, it can help you to lose some weight. They are low in calories but contain enough fiber to keep you regular and make you feel fuller. Tomatoes contain lycopene as well, which are antioxidants, helpful in removing free radicals and other toxins from your system.

Oranges

Oranges are full of vitamin C, which is needed to keep your body functioning at an optimal level. However, many people avoid oranges when they are trying to burn fat because they are worried about the sugar level. Oranges do contain sugar and, if you eat too many of them and don't burn off the sugar, it can turn to fat. However, they are low in calories and high in fiber, which helps keep your glucose levels regular. To help you to lose weight, moderate how much you eat and use it as a way of curbing a craving for candy.

Oats

Oats contain fiber, which helps to boost the metabolism, although many of those who do diets like Atkins and Paleo would disagree. A bowl of oatmeal is a fabulous way to start off the day. It isn't just full of fiber; it also contains anti-oxidants and lots of other minerals. Oats are a good way of cutting cholesterol levels.

Spices

You do not need to eat bland tasteless food when you are trying to shed some pounds so get experimenting with the contents of your spice rack. Some of them contain thermo genic properties, which help to boost the metabolism, and all of them give dishes a great taste. Mustard seed goes great on an entrée and will boost your metabolism while ginger helps your digestive system. Ginseng boosts energy and black pepper can help you to burn off calories. Turmeric is good for breaking up fat.

Sweet Potatoes

These are a fantastic addition to a diet, as a replacement for normal potatoes because they contain fewer calories and can help you to feel fuller for longer. Sweet potatoes are also loaded with potassium, fiber, vitamin B6 and vitamin C, making them the perfect replacement for a food that is normally shunned by dieters everywhere.

Apples

Not many people realize just how good an apple is. They are sweet enough to be a good replacement for sweet cravings and you can easily see why they end up in desserts. They are also low in calories, low in fat and low in sodium while being high in fiber. The fiber fills you up for longer and stops you from eating in between meals, and they also help with your digestive system too. Make sure you chew and apple thoroughly to get the best out of it.

Nuts

Every diet plan in the world include nuts and they are the one food that unites the vegetarians with the meat loving paleo dieters. They come straight from the earth and a small handful of nuts, raw and organic ones like pecans, walnuts or almonds, can be a tasty and filling snack that keep soya going for a few hours. You can also chop them and add them to a salad or sprinkle them over your food. Nuts are full of good healthy fats and full of flavor.

Quinoa

Quinoa is just starting to become popular in mainstream diets and the weight loss normally happens when you switch out rice or potatoes, or other starchy sides with quinoa. You get the full benefits of a well-rounded meals with all the vitamins contained in the quinoa. It is low in calories, low GI and full of taste.

Beans

Beans are a staple part of many diets and should be included as part of your weekly menu. They help to regulate glucose levels, help with digestion because of their high fiber content and are a great replacement for high carb foods. Black beans are

Bananas

Bananas are one of the most natural foods to eat and are the subject of many research programs for their effect on weight loss. They are so easy to add in to your diet on a daily basis because they are such a versatile fruit. They can be eaten on their own, chopped up and added to oatmeal or yoghurt and are a great source of potassium, natural sugar and energy.

Pears

Pears are often dismissed from a diet but they really should be included. They are full of flavor, and contain a whole range of benefits, which are great for weight loss. They help you to feel fuller for longer and they are different in consistency to apples and other fruits, which makes their fiber content more effective than others are. They can be eaten as they are, chopped up or cooked.

Pine Nuts

Pine nuts include a phytonutrient that can help to suppress the appetite, which means you can ditch the cost of buying expensive diet pills that are full of chemicals to do the same thing. They are tiny and they are crunchy so you can eat a lot without worrying about the effect of them and without ruining your weight loss efforts. These are one food you can binge on without any trouble.

Mushrooms

You won't see the benefits if you switch pepperoni for mushrooms on your next pizza but if you start increasing the amount you are eating, along with a range of other healthier foods, you will see a difference, because they are low in calories and high in vitamins. Don't be boring though; try all different ones from the supermarket and enjoy a range of textures, flavors and other great benefits.

Lentils

Lentils are another food that is gaining in popularity and are not just for a vegetarian diet. They contain fiber, which helps your digestive system keep your blood sugar from spiking and help you to feel fuller for longer. They are also full of protein and help to keep cholesterol levels down as well as helping the body to process carbohydrates better.

Hot Peppers

Jalapenos, chipotles and habaneros peppers are excellent weight loss foods while adding a healthy kick to the flavor of a dish. Instead of ruining your stomach lining like some believe, these will actually help to protect your stomach and prevent ulcers by killing off the bad bacteria.

Broccoli

Broccoli is one of the best superfoods. Not only are they full of anti-oxidants, they are also jam packed with nutrients and fiber. They fill you up quickly and keep your digestive system clear which makes you feel so much better. Add spices or peppers to it to give it more flavor. Broccoli with a sprinkling of turmeric has been proven to keep prostate cancer at bay as well as help you lose weight.

Organic Lean Meats

Lean meats contain all of the protein you need without the fat levels but, if you are looking to lose weight, go for organic meats.

With normal meats, the animals are pumped full of growth hormones, antibiotics and other nasty things which all end up in what you get on your plate and can slow down your weight loss. Organic meat do not contain any more nutrients than normal meat but this is a case of what it doesn't contain that makes it better. If organic is not n supply, look for grass-fed or all-natural brands.

Cantaloupe Melon

There are those who say that eating a cantaloupe burns off more calories than it contains but that is still up for debate. Whatever the outcome, it is a great food for helping to lose weight because, while it is sweet, it is low in calories, contains fiber and helps keep you moving. It is good on its own, in a fruit salad or even in a smoothie with other fruits and vegetables. Cantaloupe melon can also help to keep your skin looking great.

Spinach

Spinach is so often left lying on the plate but it is a fantastic food for health and weight loss. It is full of antioxidants, vitamins and minerals and is good to eat in a number of ways. Cook it, eat it raw in a salad, however you want. It adds bulk without adding calories. Try to go for organic and buy in bulk if you buy fresh because you can freeze it for a later date.

Green Tea

Green tea is full of antioxidants and can help you to burn off fat. This is because green tea contains catechins, which help your body to start burning off more calories and well as fat. It isn't processed like so many other teas, and is packed with antioxidants and phytonutrients that make it one of the superstar super foods.

Cinnamon

Cinnamon is one of the most powerful spices and is no longer just used for cooking. Instead, you can get the benefits from cinnamon by adding a teaspoon a day into your diet. It works by regulating your blood sugar levels, which also plays a big part in the way you are feeling throughout the day. Low blood sugar levels are indicated by a sluggish heavy feeling. Keeping your sugar levels even can also help to stop cravings. One good way is to have a drink of honey and cinnamon in hot water every day.

Asparagus

Asparagus plays a big role in weight loss with lots of different benefits and each benefit plays a specific role in weight loss. Asparagus helps to eliminate toxins from the body, helps with the digestion process and leaves the good bacteria thriving in your gut. It also has loads of vitamins, minerals and antioxidants. It tastes nice and can also be boosted with spices and seasonings.

Avocado

Avocado is a great slimming aid and contain loads of healthy fats. They were avoided for a long time because of that fat content, at a time when fat was given the label of being evil but we now know that not all fats are bad and that god fats can help to burn fat. Add avocado to salads, sandwiches, eat them as they are or make your own guacamole with them.

Peanut Butter

Peanut butter contains good fats that help to burn fat but do go for organic peanut butter as it doesn't contain any of them extra salt and sugar and tat standard peanut butter contains. It can be eaten as part of a smoothie or a piece of celery dipped in peanut butter makes a great filling snack. You can also have almond butter but it is more expensive.

Salmon

Salmon, like other fish, contains a high level of omega 3 and this is one thing that is sorely lacking in many diets today. It may be classed as a fatty fish but it is not high in saturated fats, which are the bad fats and the omega 3 content makes it better than anything else. You would need to add this in gradually to see how your body takes to it so start with once a week. If you get on with it, increase that and look around for some great tasting salmon recipes.

Apple Cider Vinegar

Go for raw organic apple cider vinegar because it contains enzymes that help your digestive system and can help with weight loss over time. The recommended way is to add it to filtered or distilled water and drink it before you eat; this helps your food to be properly digested so that your body gets all the goodness from the nutrients instead of wasting them. It can also help suppress the appetite so drink it if you find yourself hungry between meals.

Greek Yoghurt

Greek yoghurt is healthier than any other yoghurt because it is full of proteins and has a lower sugar content than normal yoghurt. You don't have to use it as a substitute for normal yoghurt though; you can use it in place of sour cream, cutting down fat and calories and you can also experiment with baking, using it in place of other fats and oils. This could take a bit of trial and error to get it right though.

Olive Oil

Olive oil is a much healthier oil than vegetable or seed oils and it can be used in a variety of ways. Not only can you add it to salads, either on its own or as part of a salad dressing, you can also use it for cooking in.

Blueberries

Blueberries are excellent for fat loss, not just weight. They help to break down sugars and fats in the body as well as tasting amazing. You can use them to add flavor to any meal and they also go well with other fruits – just skip the cream and sugar! Add them to yoghurt or oatmeal for a tasty breakfast or snack.

Turkey Breast

Turkey breast is good for those moments when you are hungry and feel as though you are going to cave in. It is a good source of lean protein and is popular on low or no carb diets. It is a god meat to eat if you are strength training and building up muscle, as well as being able to boost your metabolism.

Flax Seeds

Flax seed can be sprinkled on just about anything you want and it is a better option than sugar. It contains healthy doses of fiber, omega 3 and helps to keep you feeling fuller for longer. The essential fatty acids contained in flax seed helps to boost metabolism and lower bad cholesterol levels.

Use Fresh and Organic

Use fresh ingredients wherever possible and stick to organic. Processed foods are lower in antioxidants and have little weight loss power left in them. Organic foods are best because they don't contain the chemicals and have not been genetically modified.

You can make soups and smoothies out of some of the ingredients on this list and this is a great way to get the benefits without eating a plate of raw food. Soup is excellent for weight loss and is helps with the digestion process and you can put lots of different foods together in the same soup for a real fat busting meal that is packed full of vitamins. You can have the soup as a starter or as a meal on its own. It is also much easier to digest than some foods.

Nicholas Bjorn

Chapter 4 - The Top 20 Superfoods You Should be Eating

Everyone wants to be healthy and fit. There are many ways to stay healthy and fit, but all of them circle back to two things: exercise and diet. Nowadays, people find it difficult to follow a diet routine and an exercise regime. But if you want to stay healthy, there are no alternatives to these two options. Almost every day, we are introduced to a new form of exercise or diet routine. One such new (but really old) introduction to the world of diet is 'superfoods.'

Superfoods have become really popular nowadays thanks to the publicity they have received in recent times. There are many types of superfoods, most of them being plant-based, but there are also many superfoods that are dairy or fish-based. All these foods contain high amounts of nutrients. Some commonly found superfoods include salmon, kale, apples, blueberries, etc.

There exists no specific definition of superfoods. They are not a separate food group. Rather, superfoods are foods that contain high amounts of nutrients and are generally good for the health of your heart. Most of the superfoods contain a variety of nutrients, including protein, fats, vitamins, and essential minerals. They also contain many different antioxidants, which make them effective against cancer and similar diseases.

Many superfoods also contain a high amount of healthy fats, which are great for the health of your heart. They are also good for the health of your cardiovascular system. Many superfoods are also effective against digestive problems as well. They contain high amounts of phytochemicals that have many health benefits. Phytochemicals provide foods their deep color and taste. Adding superfoods to your day-to-day diet can help you a lot. It can bring in a lot of positive changes in your lifestyle. It can help you become fit and healthy.

In this chapter, let us have a look at twenty important superfoods that you can incorporate into your daily meals. Almost all of these superfoods are easily available on the market. Most of them are quite affordable. They are also versatile, and you can make a variety of recipes with them.

Broccoli

Broccoli is considered to be one of the healthiest vegetables as it is packed with nutrients. It contains a high amount of fiber and is rich in antioxidants as well. These properties of broccoli allow it to fight cancer. Its high antioxidant content is good for the repair of body cells and tissues. It also contains high amounts of minerals and vitamins. Broccoli is also great for the cardiovascular system and immune system. It has anti-inflammatory properties, which makes it an overall healthy vegetable. Along with its high fiber content, it is low in fats, which makes it best for people who are trying to lose weight.

Broccoli, along with other cruciferous vegetables, can reduce the growth of cancer cells. Broccoli can also reduce the blood sugar levels and is thus a boon for diabetics. Broccoli can also prevent (and reduce) cardiovascular tissue damage.

As said above, broccoli contains a high amount of fiber, which is great for digestive health. It makes bowel movements regular and smooth. Dark green vegetables such as broccoli contain a lot of nutrients that can prevent the signs of aging. One such nutrient is sulforaphane. Sulforaphane is also good for the health of the brain.

Broccoli contains a high amount of vitamin C. Vitamin C is good for the immune system. It is also good for oral health and can keep your teeth healthy. Broccoli is also good for your bones as it contains high amounts of phosphorous, calcium, and vitamin K. According to some studies, broccoli can even control joint disorders.

Broccoli is a highly recommended food for pregnant or lactating women. Broccoli is rich in nutrients, which ensures the healthy development of the fetus. It helps lactating women stay healthy. It is high in folate, which is great for the health of new mothers.

Broccoli can also control inflammation and boost immune power. It can also regulate blood sugar levels. Thus it is clear that broccoli is a superfood that can help you get healthy and fit. There are various ways of consuming broccoli. To avoid repetition, use different methods every time you cook broccoli.

Avocado

Avocado is a green, pear-shaped fruit that is often referred to as an "alligator pear." It is prized for its healthy fats, fiber, and various important nutrients. There are many types of avocado that vary in shape and color — from pear-shaped to round and green to black.

Avocados have become a highly popular food and ingredient today. They are consumed in a variety of forms and are often the main ingredient in salads, dips, shakes, etc. They are rich in vitamins- especially vitamin B, potassium, and folic acid. Another aspect that makes avocados great for health is that it allows the body to absorb nutrients effectively. This means that avocados help you to absorb the nutrients provided by other food in a more efficient manner. This is especially true in the case of carotenoids, which is an essential cancer-fighting compound.

Avocados contain high amounts of monounsaturated fatty acids, such as oleic acids. This allows them to control and manage cholesterol levels. Oleic acid is also good for preventing breast cancer.

Avocados are full of potassium, which is good for the health of the heart and bones. It can prevent many heart diseases and disorders and can also prevent stroke. It is also good for digestion and is often used for 'detox' process. Along with potassium, avocados also contain high amounts of vitamin C, B6, and D, along with manganese, and riboflavin. All these components work together to improve your immune system. They are also a good source of vitamins A and E, which can prevent cancer to a certain extent.

Another aspect that makes avocados great is that they are rich in omega-3. It reduces the risk of heart diseases and disorder and is good for your arteries. They also contain high amounts of lecithin, a type of fatty acid that is crucial for healthy nervous tissues.

Avocados are full of fiber as well. Fiber is essential for digestive health, and it can also help you lose weight. Fiber satiates you and thus prevents you from eating unnecessary and empty calories. According to various surveys, people who eat avocados regularly are comparatively healthier than those who don't. They also have a lower risk of developing metabolic diseases. Avocados contain high amounts of lutein and zeaxanthin. These antioxidants are good for the health of your eyes and optic nerves. They can also help you prevent cataract and macular degeneration.

Avocados are great for people who want to lose weight. It can help you keep full for a long time. Avocados are low in carbs and thus can help you lose weight efficiently. Incorporating avocados in your daily diet is easy as it is tasty and easy to use. You can use avocados in various forms, including avocado butter, shakes, salad, toast, etc.

Sweet Potato

Sweet potato is a delicious and nutrient-rich vegetable that is known for its distinctive sweet flavor. It is a highly versatile and healthful vegetable that is readily available in the market. Although people confuse sweet potato with yam all the time, both of them are different. Sweet potato is one of the most easily available and nutrient-rich superfoods. It contains high amounts of beta-carotene, which is a great antioxidant.

Sweet potato also contains high amounts of vitamin A. This vitamin is essential for the health of our bones, skin, immune system, eyes, and reproductive system as well. Sweet potato also has nutrients that can help you prevent cancer. It also contains high amounts of vitamin C, which is great for people who have asthma or arthritis. It can also help people who have diabetes as it has a very low glycemic index, which means it does not have a significant effect on blood glucose levels.

As said above, sweet potato is sweet in taste and is a starchy root vegetable that is grown all around the globe. This tube is available in various sizes, shapes, and colors. They contain high amounts of fiber, which makes them a great food for people who are trying to lose weight. They also increase the number of good gut bacteria that is good for the digestive system.

Sweet potatoes contain high amounts of different antioxidants. These antioxidants are helpful against various types of cancers. For instance, sweet potato contains anthocyanin, an antioxidant that is well known for slowing down the growth of cancerous cells of cancers affecting bladder, colon, breast, and the stomach. Sweet potatoes are also a rich source of beta-carotene, which is good for optical health.

Sweet potatoes are extremely versatile and can be used like regular potatoes. There are many different ways of cooking sweet potatoes. They can be boiled, roasted, baked, fried pan-cooked, or steamed. It is possible to consume them with skin or without skin as well. If you like eating chips, try eating sweet potato chips. These chips are healthier than regular chips. As sweet potatoes are naturally sweet, they go well with many different flavors. You can make sweet as well as savory dishes with sweet potatoes.

considered being the best source of dietary omega 3. Other, considerably cost-effective fish such as herring roe and sardines too contain omega-3, but salmon contain the highest amounts.

Fish is a really good source of omega 3 as they provide long-chain polyunsaturated fatty acids. These acids are as follows: Eicosapentaenoic and docosahexaenoic acid (EPA and DHA). Such combinations are only found in seafood and marine algae or seaweed. Terrain plants provide short-chain omega-3 alpha-linolenic acid (ALA). The human body can utilize ALA to synthesize EPA and DHA, but getting them directly from the source is always better as it reduces the work and energy required. For instance, one 4 oz portion of cooked salmon can provide approximately 2000 mg of omega-3s.

The human body needs L-tryptophan (an amino acid) to make melatonin. This acid is found in abundance in salmon. This is why people who eat salmon regularly rarely face any sleep-related problems. A 4 oz serving of salmon contains approximately 250–400 mg of L-tryptophan.

The vitamin B family is necessary for the body as these vitamins are used to regulate energy metabolism and enhance tissue formation as well. Salmon contains a lot of vitamin Bs, including B2, B3, B6, and B12. If you are a pescatarian, then eating salmon is one of the best ways to get vitamin B12. A 4 oz piece of salmon contains 5.7 mcg of B12 or 236% of the recommended daily intake.

Salmon also contains high amounts of minerals, such as phosphorus and calcium. These minerals are good for the health of your teeth and bones. It also contains other trace materials such as selenium, which is a great antioxidant. A 4 oz serving of salmon provides 365 mg of phosphorus or 52% of the recommended daily intake.

Salmon is also a great source of protein. Salmon contains various amino acids that are essential for the health of your body. It also contains proteins such as calcitonin, which promotes healthy joints and bones.

Astaxanthin is another antioxidant that is found in abundance in salmon and similar seafood. It is a fat-soluble pigment that is red in color; this is why salmon looks so red. It also contains high amounts of carotenoids that can reduce the number of free radicals. This is why salmon is considered to be one of the best superfoods.

Pomegranate Seeds

Pomegranate is considered to be one of the best superfoods currently available. It has been used since ancient times in the Middle East and has been celebrated for its taste and health benefits. The outer skin of the pomegranate is tough, but the insides are juicy, delicious, and blood red.

The seeds of pomegranate are slightly tart and sweet. These seeds not only help you stay healthy but also free of disease. They are a great addition to your salads as they will not only make it more colorful and healthy, but it will make your salads tasty as well.

As said earlier, pomegranates were used in Asia, India, Africa, and the Mediterranean since ancient times. In ancient times, pomegranates were used to denote fertility. It is one of the most represented fruits in art throughout the centuries.

Pomegranate was introduced to North America around a few centuries ago. It is now grown in abundance in parts of Arizona and California. All the parts of pomegranates contain immense amounts of nutrients. This is why pomegranates have become such a rage in the world of superfoods. Nowadays, pomegranates are easily available in the market in the form of juices, extracts, powders, supplements, etc. The fruits are available in abundance in supermarkets.

Pomegranates can help you lower cholesterol, which makes them great for cardiovascular and heart diseases. Pomegranates also contain high amounts of vitamin C, which provides them immense anti-inflammatory properties. Pomegranates are also potent against certain cancers and Type 2 diabetes as well. Pomegranates also contain high amounts of antioxidants, which can help to reduce high blood pressure. Pomegranate is also good for the health of your brain, arteries, and heart.

According to certain studies, if you consume around 8 oz of pomegranate juice daily, it can work wonders for your health. Pomegranate is also good for 'masculine health.' It can improve erections and can also slow down the growth of prostate cancer cells as well.

Blueberries

Blueberries are versatile fruits that can be either eaten raw and fresh or can be utilized in a variety of recipes as well. Blueberries can be used fresh or can be eaten frozen as well.

Blueberries contain high amounts of anthocyanin. This compound gives them a distinct color. It is also responsible for its numerous health benefits. Blueberries are good for the health of your heart. They are also good for your skin, hair, blood pressure, bone strength, diabetes, mental health, and cancer. One cup of blueberries can provide you with 24% of the daily total vitamin C requirement.

As said above, blueberries are exceptionally versatile, and they can be used in a variety of forms and in a variety of recipes as well. For instance, blueberries are often used to top salads, ice cream, yogurt, shakes, pancakes, cereals, oatmeal, and salads too. They can also be blended into syrups and smoothies. You can also add them to sweetbreads and muffins. You can make a variety of desserts with blueberries.

Blueberries also contain high amounts of vitamin K. This is why people who are on blood thinners should avoid using a lot of blueberries or should consult their health professional before eating a lot of blueberries.

Blueberries contain many different flavonoids. Flavonoids are antioxidants that have multiple health benefits.

Eating a variety of fruits and vegetables is one of the best ways to stay healthy and tackle diseases and disorders. For instance, a lot of studies have proved the consuming blueberries can help you tackle obesity, heart problems, diabetes, and various other diseases as well. Blueberries can improve your overall health. Blueberries are also good for people who are trying to lose weight. They are also good for the health of your skin and hair.

Blueberries are often sold frozen. While freezing them ensures a long shelf life, the process removes many essential nutrients. According to a study, the amount of anthocyanin in frozen blueberries decreases rapidly, and in a couple of months, it can go down by 30-40 %. More research is required regarding this. But it is always better to buy and eat fresh blueberries whenever you can. Try to find organic berries.

Blueberries contain a variety of minerals as well. For instance, they are rich in calcium, phosphorus, iron, magnesium, zinc, manganese, and vitamin K. All these nutrients are good for the health of your bones. If you consume adequate amounts of vitamins and minerals, your bones become healthy and non-brittle. Iron and zinc are responsible for the health of your joints. Vitamin K deficiency often leads to brittle bones. This is because vitamin K improves the absorption of calcium. A low amount of vitamin K ultimately leads to a low amount of calcium.

Collagen is essential for the health of our skin. It keeps it tight, young, fresh, and healthy. Collagen needs a lot of vitamin C to perform properly. Collagen also protects the skin from various damaging factors such as pollution, the sun, and smoke. Blueberries contain high amounts of vitamin C, which enhances the potency of collagen. Thus, blueberries can help you achieve beautiful and attractive looking skin.

Blueberries contain no sodium. Excessive sodium is bad for your health, especially for your blood pressure. On the other hand, blueberries are full of calcium, potassium, and magnesium. The deficiency of these minerals can often lead to high blood pressure. Thus, blueberries can help you regulate your blood pressure.

A high fiber diet is recommended for people who have Type 1 diabetes. A high fiber diet can help to lower blood glucose levels. Similarly, people suffering from Type 2 diabetes can also benefit a lot from consuming a high fiber diet. A single cup of blueberries contains around 3.6 grams of fiber.

Blueberries are also good for the health of your heart. They contain high amounts of potassium, fiber, folate, vitamin B6, vitamin C, and phytonutrients. All these nutrients are essential for the health of your heart. Blueberries contain no cholesterol. The fiber in blueberries can reduce the amount of cholesterol present in the body already.

Homocysteine is a harmful chemical that is present in our body. A lot of homocysteine can lead to clogging and damaging blood vessels. It is extremely dangerous for the health of or heart. Blueberries contain a high amount of vitamin B6 and folate, which can prevent the buildup of homocysteine.

According to a study, it was found that women who consumed around three servings of blueberries every week showed a reduced risk of heart diseases and disorders. The various vitamins present in blueberries act as antioxidants that can tackle free radicals present in the body.

According to research, antioxidants can also prevent the growth of tumors and reduce inflammation. They can slow down the growth of cancer cells in the lungs, esophagus, mouth, pharynx, pancreas, colon, and prostate. They can also prevent endometrial cancer, as well.

Blueberries are rich in folate. Folate plays a crucial role in the repair and synthesis of DNA. Due to this, the DNA does not mutate. DNA mutations are often responsible for cancer.

Blueberries can also tackle cognitive damage, especially in women. Similar studies have proved how blueberries can improve memory and coordination. It can also help to prevent and tackle other brain-related problems.

Blueberries are also great against constipation. They are good for the health of your digestive system. They contain lots of fiber, which is good for digestion. Dietary fiber is also good for weight loss and weight management. High fiber foods lead to early satiation. This way, you do not end up consuming a lot of empty calories, making blueberries a miracle berry!

Quinoa

Quinoa has become a rage in the world of fitness and health now. Quinoa is considered one of the healthiest and nutrient-rich foods available in the market. It is a highly healthy and delicious food. It is a highly versatile and incredible food that is a great source of carbs. Many people believe that quinoa is a grain just like rice or wheat, but it is quite different than them. In fact, quinoa is not a grain at all. It is known as pseudo-grain. It is a form of seed that is highly nutritious.

Quinoa is one of the most nutrient-dense carbs available today. It has around six grams of proteins per cup. It is also the only carb source that contains all nine essential amino acids. Along with this, quinoa is a complete protein. It also contains a high amount of lysine. Lysine is an amino acid that is necessary for healing and repairing muscles. This is why many gym rats generally include quinoa in their diet.

Quinoa also has many other benefits, such as it is full of various minerals and vitamins. It is a rich source of copper, iron, phosphorus, and manganese. Manganese and copper control free radicals and are good for the health of bones and teeth. Phosphorous and iron play an integral role in the creation of energy. Then it can also help against the development of cancer cells. Another point that makes quinoa really great is that it is

Stop Dieting

full of fiber. Each serving contains around 2.5 grams of fiber. Fiber is great for people who are trying to lose weight. It satiates you and keeps you feeling full for a long time. This way, you do not consume random, useless calories. Fiber is also good for the health of your digestive tract. It is also good for diabetics as it improves the function of insulin.

Nowadays, there are many different recipes of quinoa available online. While North America is trying to grow quinoa locally, a lot of quinoa is still imported from South America. Due to the increasing demands of quinoa, it has become a priced commodity. But the price is definitely worth the health benefits of the product. This is why people are still buying quinoa in abundance.

Nowadays, quinoa is available in a variety of forms. For instance, you can now buy quinoa cereal, pasta, flour, cookies, etc. It is an extremely versatile food product and can be used in a variety of recipes. You can make delicious desserts, cookies, granola bars, cakes, side dishes, breakfast foods, shakes, etc. from quinoa. It is easy to use, which is why many people now try to incorporate it into their daily meals.

Quinoa is a boon for people who are allergic to gluten. It contains no gluten and is thus great for people who are on a no-gluten diet. Gluten is found in many essential grains such as rye, oats, wheat, and barley, which make them unsuitable for anyone who has celiac disease or is allergic to gluten. Quinoa is rich in nutrients and contains no gluten, which has made it really popular with the gluten-free community.

Quinoa has a slightly nutty flavor that is not at all overpowering and goes well with almost everything. It is easy to cook, and it hardly takes more than 12-15 minutes to get done. It is also popular with kids in the form of cereal and cookies.

Almonds

Almonds are not only tasty, but they are also full of nutrients. They contain high amounts of minerals, proteins, vitamins, fiber, etc. Their nutrition makes them a really healthy superfood. For instance, only a handful of almonds contain around 1/8th of our daily protein needs. Almonds are versatile, and there are multiple ways to eat them. You can eat them raw, or you can also toast them. They are often added to sweet as well as savory dishes as toppings or garnish. They are a great addition to salads as they provide a good crunch to it. Nowadays, almonds are available in a variety of forms, including chopped almonds, peeled almonds, slivered almonds, sliced almonds, almond flakes, almond flour, almond oil, almond milk, and almond butter. Almond is known as a nut, but it is actually a seed full of nutrients.

Almond trees are one of the earliest plants that human beings cultivated. Archaeologists have found evidence showcasing that people in Jordan domesticated almond trees around 5000 years ago. Almonds are full of fats, but they are full of unsaturated fats. Unsaturated fats are healthy and essential for the body. They do not increase LDL or low-density lipoprotein. LDL is often known as "bad" cholesterol.

According to the AHA or American Heart Association, moderate amounts of unsaturated fats can improve your cholesterol levels. Almonds contain no cholesterol. According to a study published in 2005 says that almonds also contain high amounts of vitamin E. Vitamin E is an essential antioxidant that can stop the oxidization process that is responsible for the clogging of arteries. Along with this, another study conducted in 2018 found the same results. According to this study, almonds can help to increase or maintain the levels of HDL or high-density lipoprotein or "good" cholesterol. According to this study, people are recommended to consume at least 45 grams of almonds a day for cardiovascular health.

According to a 2015 study, almonds can help against cancer as well. The study says that almonds can reduce the risk of breast cancer by about two to three times. Peanuts and walnuts, too, were found to be helpful against breast cancer.

In another study conducted in 2011, around 20 people suffering from Type 2 diabetes were observed. They were asked to eat 60 g of almonds every day for 12 weeks. It was found that the almonds improved their blood lipids, blood sugar levels, and fat levels as well.

One oz of almonds contains around 76. 5 mg of magnesium on average. This is around 20-24% of the total daily requirement of a healthy adult. While magnesium supplements are a great way to tackle deficiency, healthy people can eat almonds to avoid becoming deficient.

Almonds contain high amounts of fibers, proteins, and healthy fats. They are low in carbs. These factors make them great for people who are trying to lose weight. According to a study conducted in 2015, people who eat almonds as morning snacks eat fewer calories throughout the day. This is because almonds contain fiber, which helps you stay satiated for a long time. This is why almonds are often a staple ingredient of breakfast cereals and muesli.

Almonds are also a rich source of vitamin K, manganese, calcium, copper, zinc, and protein. All these are responsible for good and healthy bones.

Beet Roots

Beetroot is a delicious, healthy, and great looking vegetable that is packed with nutrients. Beet leaves are healthy as well. Beetroot has been used since ancient times for various medical purposes. For instance, it was once upon a time used to treat fevers, skin issues, constipation, etc.

Beetroot contains high amounts of folate and iron. Folate is naturally occurring folic acid, which is good for your health. It also contains high amounts of magnesium, nitrates, betaine, betacyanin, and many other antioxidants that are good for health. According to recent studies, it has been proven that beetroots can also help to lower blood pressure and can prevent dementia as well. It is great for gym rats as it increases stamina.

As said above, beetroot contains high amounts of nitrates. Nitrates are converted into nitric oxide by our bodies. This chemical can lower blood pressure. According to studies, beetroot can moderately control blood pressure; however, more study is necessary. It is still considered to be great for the health of your heart and cardiovascular system.

Another study conducted in 2013 showed the relation between beetroots and improved exercise and performance. According to this study, beetroot can improve activity inactive as well as inactive individuals. But elite athletes showed little to no change.

According to a study conducted in 2010, beetroot juice can enhance the flow of blood in the brain. It is also good for the skin and hair and has many cosmetic benefits.

Beetroot has a distinct color and flavor. It is recommended to consume it raw, but you can also cook it according to the recipe. It is a great addition to salads as it provides taste, color, and crunch. Beetroot juice is another common form in which beetroot can be consumed with ease.

Kale

Kale is considered one of the healthiest leafy vegetables. It contains high amounts of nutrients and is really great for people who are trying to lose weight. Kale contains many medicinal properties as well. Kale is highly versatile, and it can be had in many different forms. It is easy to incorporate in daily meals. It can be eaten raw, fried, or it can be made into soups and salads as well. Thus, kale is one of the best superfoods currently available.

Kale is a member of the cabbage family. Like other cruciferous vegetables, such as broccoli, Brussels sprouts, and cauliflower, kale too is extremely healthy and nutritious. There are many different varieties of kale available in the market. Green and purple varieties are the most popular. The shape of leaves of kale varieties varies a lot. Some have plain leaves, while others have curved and rounded leaves. Curly Kale or Scots Kale is a popular variety of kale that has curly leaves and a stark green color.

Kale is extremely rich in nutrients. A single cup contains high amounts of minerals such as calcium, manganese, potassium, copper, and magnesium. It also contains high amounts of vitamins such as A, K, C, B6. A single cup of kale contains around 6 grams of carbs, 3 grams of proteins, and only 33 calories. Kale contains little to no fat, which makes it great for people who are trying to lose weight. Kale is considered to be one of the most nutrient-dense foods in the world.

Kale is rich in antioxidants like other green leafy vegetables. It contains high amounts of beta-carotene, Quercetin, and Kaempferol. It also contains high amounts of vitamin C, which is good for your immune system. In fact, a cup of kale contains more vitamin C than an orange!

Kale contains high amounts of bile acids, such as sequestrants, which can control your cholesterol level. Thus, kale is really great for the health of your heart and cardiovascular system as well.

Cancer is an extremely terrible disease that can wreak havoc in a person's life. Kale contains many components that can fight cancer efficiently.

Kale contains high amounts of minerals and can thus prevent mineral deficiency. Spinach is another green leafy vegetable that is full of nutrients, but when compared to kale, spinach falls short. Kale is not only rich in minerals, but it is also low in oxalate.

People who are trying to lose weight are often worried about their diet and what to eat and what not to eat. Kale is definitely a great choice for anyone who is trying to lose weight. It is low in calories but can still keep you satiated for a long time.

Spinach

Spinach is a great leafy vegetable that contains high amounts of nutrients. It is dark, leafy, and contains very few calories. It is good for your skin, bones, hair, and heart. It also contains high amounts of iron, protein, minerals, and vitamins. Spinach can help you to control blood sugar levels, improve bone health, and can also lower the risk of cancer significantly. It also contains a variety of minerals that are good for your health.

Spinach has been used by many different cultures since ancient times. It is a staple food of middle-eastern, Mediterranean, and Southeast Asian cultures. It is versatile and can be added to almost any food. It has its own distinct flavor, but it is not overpowering and thus can be mixed with other ingredients with ease. Spinach is also cheap and easy to cook. There are many different ways of cooking spinach, but you can also eat it raw. Spinach is really good for reducing oxidative stress. It is also good for blood pressure levels and optical health as well.

Spinach contains high amounts of insoluble fiber, which is good for weight loss and digestion. It also contains high amounts of lutein, kaempferol, quercetin, nitrates, and zeaxanthin, which are all good for your health.

Spinach contains high amounts of vitamin K1, so people who suffer from kidney stones should avoid it. It is also not recommended for people who are on blood thinners. Other than these people, everyone can consume spinach.

Green Tea

Green tea is a great beverage that contains many different nutrients. It has many health benefits and properties due to the way it is prepared and processed. To make black tea, the tea leaves are fermented, which gives it a distinct taste and color. In the case of green tea, the leaves are steamed. Due to this, the tea leaves do not lose a lot of nutrients and taste. This is why green tea is extremely rich in antioxidants.

Green tea is known to prevent or slow down the growth of cancer. It fights the battle against cancer on all fronts. For instance, it protects the DNA against any damage. It also attacks the cancerous cells. It can even shut down crucial molecules that are responsible for the development of cancer.

According to recent Swedish research, green tea also stops the formation of new blood vessels. These vessels are responsible for spreading tumors.

Green tea can also reduce and repair the damage caused to the liver due to alcohol. It is also good against various diseases, including Parkinson's and rheumatoid arthritis. It also prevents cholesterol from choking blood vessels. Women who drink green tea regularly have better bones than those who don't. Thus, green tea also reduces the risk of osteoporosis in women.

Green tea is full of nutrients, such as antioxidants that are great for the body. These are responsible for enhanced brain function, reduced risk of cancer, and enhanced fat loss as well.

Green tea also contains small amounts of caffeine that can keep you awake for a long time. It also acts as a stimulant and is good for the health of your brain. While the amount of caffeine present in green tea is lower than the amount present in coffee, it is still potent enough to give you efficient results.

Green tea also contains important amino acids, such as L-theanine. This amino acid works in combination with caffeine to improve brain function. Green tea can also boost your

The type of fiber that is present in apple acts as food for bacteria. These good gut bacteria are essential for digestive health. They are also helpful in the case of heart problems, obesity, and Type 2 diabetes. Apples also contain many different nutrients that can fight cancer efficiently.

Apples also contain high amounts of anti-inflammatory compounds and antioxidants. They can help the regular immune system. These antioxidants are also good for the health of your bones. Apples are also great for your memory as they reduce wear and tear of neurotransmitters.

Flax Seeds

Flax seeds are tiny, but they contain high amounts of nutrients. They are full of omega-3, fiber, fatty acids, antioxidants, lignans, and many different varieties of vitamin B. Only a couple of teaspoons of flax seeds per day can provide you a lot of nutrients and can keep you healthy and fit. Incorporating flax seeds in your daily diet is easy as they can be added to literally any food, including salads, shakes, desserts, etc. Flax seeds and flaxseed oil have both been used for cooking for a long time. A lot of records regarding flax seeds have been found throughout the world.

Flax seeds come from the flowers of the flax plant. They are slightly larger than sesame seeds. They are normally available in shades such as dark brown and golden tan. They are flat and shiny. The seeds have a slightly nutty and earthy flavor, but their flavor often gets overpowered by other flavors when they are used in other dishes.

While flax seeds contain a multitude of nutrients, they are celebrated for being rich in lignans, omega 3, and fiber.

Flax seeds are great for vegetarians and vegans. Normally the best source for omega 3 is salmon, but vegans can get a lot of omega 3 from flaxseed. Flax seeds contain high amounts of ALA, which is a form of omega 3. ALA is good for the health of your heart, and it can also reduce the risk of stroke.

Along with ALA, flax seeds also contain high amounts of lignans. Lignans are a group of ingredients that are highly potent antioxidants. They can help to prevent breast and prostate cancer. They can also slow down the development of other cancers as well.

Flax seeds are great for people who suffer from digestive problems or are trying to lose weight. As flax seeds are full of fiber, they can improve your digestion. A high amount of fiber can also lower cholesterol and can improve the health of your heart as well. Flaxseeds also contain a high amount of insoluble fiber. Insoluble fiber can lower your blood sugar levels significantly — this why doctors often recommend diabetic patients to incorporate flax seeds in their diet.

Flax seeds are also great for people who are trying to lose weight. Flax seeds contain a high amount of fiber, which keeps you full for a long time.

Incorporating flax seeds into your diet is easy. You can either consume raw flax seeds or roasted flax seeds. The easiest way to eat flax seeds is by using them in shakes and salads. You can also consume spoonfuls of flax seeds twice daily. Flaxseed oil/gel is also great for the health of your hair and skin.

Oats

Oats have become really popular in modern times. They are high in nutrients that are available almost everywhere. They are extremely beneficial for our health. Oats are generally 100% whole grains that undergo a very low amount of processing. They contain high amounts of minerals, vitamins, and fiber. They also contain high amounts of beta-glucan. This is a soluble fiber that is good for lower cholesterol reabsorption. Oats also contain low amounts of sodium and a good amount of protein, which makes it great for people trying to lose weight.

According to the FDA review, oats can reduce LDLs, i.e., the lower serum cholesterol levels. This is a result of beta-glucan. This soluble fiber has made oats really popular among masses, especially among people who are trying to lose weight. While oats do help you to lose weight, they are not a 'one-time magic' solution that works instantly. You do need to combine oats with other methods of weight loss.

Oats are low in calories and contain high amounts of proteins and fiber. This makes them great for people trying to lose weight. They contain high amounts of potassium, magnesium, zinc, manganese, copper, thiamine, selenium, and pantothenic acid. They also contain high amounts of phytonutrients such as phytoestrogens, polyphenols, lignins, vitamin R, and protease inhibitors.

According to studies, if individuals who have high cholesterol consume even 3 grams of oat fiber every day (i.e., a bowl of oatmeal), their cholesterol levels can go down by 8-23 percent. Even a 1 percent drop is good for the heart and reduces the risk of developing heart disease. Thus, oats are really good for people who are at risk of developing heart problems.

Oats contain a lot of nutrients that make them exceptionally good for people who are trying to eat healthily and stay fit. They are good for your immune system and can help you tackle a lot of diseases and disorders as well. Oats are available with ease almost everywhere in the world. They are a staple ingredient in many baked goods. Almost all restaurants and breakfast places feature different kinds of oatmeal on their menu.

As said above, there are many different varieties of oats available in the market. Steel-cut oats can bring a lot of texture and flavor to otherwise plain and bland foods.

Oats are extremely versatile, and there are various methods of cooking and eating them. The easiest way to consume oats is in the form of cereals or oatmeal, but you can also consume oats in the form of cookies, cakes, shakes, salads, etc. Oats do not have a strong flavor profile and thus can be mixed with anything.

Hemp Seeds

It may come as a surprise, but it is true, hemp seeds are really good for your health. The scientific name of hemp seeds is Cannabis Sativa. Nowadays, thanks to research, people have realized that hemp seeds are indeed a superfood. They contain high amounts of nutrients that are really good for your body. Many people call hemp seeds to be the most nutritious food available for consumption. Hemp seeds are great for weight loss as they contain a high amount of fiber. They can help you stay full for a long time. They can also reduce your hunger pangs and thus ultimately control your weight. Eating hemp seeds is easy; just add a couple of teaspoons to your morning meal. Eating hemp seeds in the morning will help you stay satiated for a long time throughout the day.

Hemp seeds can be eaten raw, whole, toasted, or roasted. Nowadays, they are also available in various flavors to make them more palatable. You can use these seeds in various ways. You can also use the oil prepared from these seeds. The leftover stuff remaining after extracting oil from hemp seeds is quite nutrient-rich as well. Hemp is as healthy as any green vegetable. The health benefits of hemp and hemp seeds have now been proven by science as well.

Hemp seeds can efficiently reduce the risk of heart disease. Heart diseases and disorders are the two leading causes of death all around the world. According to research, hemp seeds can reduce the risk of developing heart diseases and disorders. Hemp seeds contain high amounts of amino acids. These acids produce nitric oxide in the body. This nitric oxide is good for the health of your blood vessels as it relaxes them and thus lowers and regulates your blood pressure. This, in turn, reduces the risk of heart disorders.

Omega 6, omega 3, and amino acids are essential for a healthy immune system. Hemp seeds are rich sources of these three nutrients and are thus great for your immune system. Amino acids are also good for the health of your skin. Hemp seed oil can work wonders for all your skin problems, including signs of aging, dark spots, acne, etc.

Hemp seeds are a boon for women suffering from menopause and PMS. It can effectively tackle the symptoms of PMS. According to studies, the hormone prolactin causes the symptoms associated with PMS. Hemp seeds contain a high amount of gamma linoleum acid, which can tackle prolactin by producing prostaglandin el.

Hemp seeds also contain a high amount of fiber. They contain both insoluble and soluble fiber in an 80:20 ratio. This makes hemp seeds really good for your digestive health.

Hemp seeds do not contain any trans fats, which makes them great for people who are trying to lose weight. Thus, including hemp seeds in your regular diet will help you become fit, healthy, and young. If you do not like the taste of hemp seeds, try using the flavored ones.

Goji Berries

Goji berries have become one of the most celebrated superfoods now. They are reddish-orange berries that grow on the wolfberry plant. These plants are native to China. They are kind of tart but also have an inherent sweetness. Goji berries are more popular for their health benefits. They contain high amounts of antioxidants and a variety of nutrients as well.

Ancient Chinese medicine schools have been using goji berries for thousands of years for a variety of ailments and problems. Recently, goji berries and their immense health benefits have been introduced to the western world, which is why they have become a staple in health food stores.

Goji berries contain a high amount of vitamin C, even more than oranges. It also contains a high amount of selenium, calcium, iron, potassium, and zinc.

Goji berries also contain a high number of carotenoids, such as beta-carotene. It is good for the health of your eyes and optical nerves. It also contains a high amount of fiber, which is good for your digestive system. Goji berries can reduce fatigue and stress by giving your energy boosts. They contain a high amount of melatonin, which makes them great for people who suffer from insomnia or other sleep-related problems.

Goji berries are also rich in protein. They contain around 12-14% protein. They are the right combination of taste and health. In the west, these berries are generally available in dried form. High quality dried berries are soft and fleshy.

Goji berries are versatile, and there are many different ways you can use them. Some people prefer to eat them right out of the bag. They can also be mixed with other dried fruits, seeds, and nuts. You can also add them to smoothies and shakes. Some people also like to toss some berries in their salads. This makes the salad look and taste good.

Coconut

Coconut is a great superfood that can help you become fit and healthy. It is a versatile fruit that can be used in a variety of forms. Some of the most common forms include dried coconut, raw coconut meat, coconut oil, coconut water, coconut milk, etc. Coconuts have been grown and used since ancient times in various tropical regions around the world. Now they are gaining rapid popularity all over the world thanks to their immense culinary versatility and numerous health benefits.

While other fruits are full of carbs, coconut contains high amounts of fats. They are also a rich source of protein, vitamins, and minerals. Coconut contains a high amount of manganese, which is good for the health of your bones. It also metabolizes proteins, cholesterol, and carbs efficiently.

Coconuts are also rich in iron and copper. They also contain selenium. Selenium is an essential antioxidant that keeps your cells healthy.

Coconut contains high amounts of MCT or medium-chain triglycerides. Our body uses these fats for instant energy and does not store them. Thus, coconut is good for people who are trying to lose weight.

Coconut is also great for the health of your heart. It was found that people who live on Polynesian islands rarely get heart diseases and disorders. This is because their diet is rich in coconuts. According to certain studies, if you consume coconut oil, it may help you to reduce belly fat. This is especially great for people who are trying to lose weight. According to studies, coconut oil can also reduce cholesterol levels.

Coconut contains high amounts of fiber and fat but a low amount of carbs. This combination is great for your blood sugar levels. It can reduce your blood sugar levels efficiently.

Coconuts contain arginine. Arginine is an essential amino acid that improves pancreatic activity. It plays an important role in the regulation of blood sugar levels. Eating coconut also affects the beta cells present in the pancreas, which are responsible for the production of insulin.

Due to the high fiber content of coconut meat, you can also lose weight and stay satiated for a long time.

Coconuts are full of various antioxidants. Most of these antioxidants are phenolic compounds such as caffeic acid, gallic acid, salicylic acid, p-coumaric acid, etc. All these acids are good for the health of your body as they tackle free radicals.

It also contains a high number of polyphenols, which reduces the oxidation of LDL. Oxidized LDL leads to the formation of plaque in arteries.

Coconuts are extremely versatile, and they can be eaten in a variety of ways. Shaved or flaked coconuts are great for savory dishes. Shaved coconut is a great addition to rice, stews, soups, curries, etc. Certain brands of shaved coconut contain sugar, so it is best to avoid them if you want to lose weight.

Shredded coconut is great for desserts and baked goods. Raw coconut can add a really brilliant tropical flavor to any dish. If you are allergic to gluten, then you can replace wheat flour with coconut flour. This flower is also suitable for Paleo diet followers.

Coconut oil can be used for cooking, frying, baking, and roasting as well.

Garlic

Garlic has been used for its taste enhancing and medicinal properties since ancient times. Hippocrates, the father of modern medicine, used to prescribe garlic for a variety of ailments. Now modern science has confirmed and proved its health benefits.

Garlic is a member of the onion or Allium family. The members of this family, such as onions, shallots, etc. contain a lot of sulfur compounds that are responsible for the health benefits. One such compound is allicin. Along with allicin, other compounds that make garlic healthy include diallyl disulfide and s-allyl cysteine. Garlic is great for weight loss as it contains a very low number of calories. One clove of raw garlic has:

- 2% of daily manganese

- 2% of daily vitamin B6

- 1% of daily vitamin C

- 1% of daily selenium

- 0.06 grams of fiber

It also contains moderate amounts of copper, calcium, potassium, iron, phosphorus, and vitamin B1.

It contains only 4.5 calories and 1 gram of carbs. It also contains around 0.2 grams of protein. Garlic is good for the health of your immune system. It is effective against the common cold as well. It is also used to treat cough and sore throat.

Garlic is supposed to be great for the health of your heart as well. It is good for hypertension and high blood pressure, as well. Garlic can also reduce the levels of cholesterol and thus reduce the risk of heart diseases. It is really effective against LDL cholesterol.

Garlic is rich in antioxidants. These antioxidants can tackle free radicals and prevent oxidative damage as well. These antioxidants can also improve your immune system. According to some sources, garlic can also target Alzheimer's and dementia as well.

Garlic can also increase your longevity. It can tackle many different infections, as well as chronic diseases. Garlic also has detoxifying effects that can prevent organ damage by getting rid of harmful chemicals from the body. Another thing that makes garlic really great for health is that it can make your bones strong. It reduces bone damage, especially in the case of women. It can reduce the occurrence of osteoporosis in women.

Garlic is a versatile food item that can be incorporated into various recipes. It goes great with bread, soups, and sauces. Garlic has a strong taste, and thus, it can make otherwise bland food taste good. Garlic can be used in a variety of forms. The most commonly used forms are cloves. It is also possible to use garlic in the form of pastes and powders. Nowadays, garlic oil is used in a lot of cuisines as well.

Garlic can cause halitosis if used improperly. It is recommended to avoid using garlic if you are allergic to it. Garlic is also not recommended for people who are on blood-thinners.

Chapter 5 – 8 Reasons Why You Are Not Losing Body Fat

Collectively, we spend years of our lives trying to shed those extra pounds of body fat but have little to no success. We go on diet after diet, our weight yo-yoing up and down and we ride on a rollercoaster that has way too much roll in it. We try to shed the fat when we are motivated but still fall apart when we see a plate of fresh warm cookies. Unfortunately, this is why so many New Year's resolutions wind up discarded and gym memberships get ignored. While we might have a common goal in mind, losing fat, it is not an easy thing to achieve satisfactorily.

If you have been playing the same game and haven't yet succeeded, you are more than likely making a couple of mistakes. Below I am going to talk about the 8 most common mistakes that people make when they are trying to lose fat:

Mistake Number 1 – You are eating too much

This might seem like an obvious on but so many people seriously do not know how many calories they are eating. A salad might seem like a low calorie option but you may actually be munching your way through 600 calories. Salad dressings, sauces, ketchups and oils are all loaded with calories that you don't always see or think about, especially if you are not a regular cook at home.

We are always told to eat less calories than we are burning but this simplifies matters too much. This would work if you, for example, ate 1500 calories worth of cheesecake every day and burned 2000 calories. But, the one thing the human body can't do is be a calculator. What matters is not how many calories but the type of calories you are eating. If you eat a diet that is made up of carbohydrates only, you won't burn any fat, whereas if you eat less of the carbs and more protein, fat and the right carbs, you are on to a winning combination for burning fat and building up muscle.

Most people find that a ratio of 40% carbs, 40% protein and 20% fat works perfectly to burn off that fat. However, that may not work for all so you will need to do your research and work out what is best for you. Some people have to reduce their carb limit even lower to be successful but, if you have to do that, boost up your good fat intake to allow your body an alternative source of energy to burn.

Mistake Number 2 – You are not eating enough protein

Protein isn't just for building and repairing your muscle tissue. Recent studies have showed that, on two groups of women who were overweight, both of whom consumed the same number of calories per day, the group that consumed 128 g protein every day lost more weight than the group who consumed just 68 g protein per day.

Protein makes you feel fuller for much longer and stops you from grazing throughout the day and from eating too much at your main meals. A high protein diet can also affect the glucose levels, blood lipids and muscle to fat ratio in the body in a positive manner. Protein is an excellent fat loss macro but you will not see instant results by adding protein shakes to your diet. Fat burning is not instant; it takes dedication and consistently following the meal plan to make a difference. What you can do is add high protein foods to your meals and cut down on the bad carbs foods – you will see the results in time.

Stop Dieting

Mistake Number 3 – You are drinking too much

You really only need to drink water. You can have tea or coffees, occasionally milk but stop the stream of sugar-filled drinks. All they are doing is undoing the good work the rest of your food is doing. One pumpkin spice latte can contain over 300 calories, and that is just in one drink! That is not doing your body any good at all – all you are doing is making your fat loss goas harder to attain.

Alcohol is also a bad call. While a beer or a glass of wine every now and again isn't going to make much difference, you must stop the binging at weekends. Alcohol is high in calories, these are stored by your body as fat, and it also causes an impairment to your judgment. Instead of eating a good healthy choice, the booze will tell you that a big pate of cheesy chips is just the right thing to eat.

Mistake Number 4 – You think that healthy foods have no calories

Everything has calories in it, regardless of how healthy it is. If you eat too much, you will struggle to shed the fat. Of course, you need to eat whole foods but eating too much organic peanut butter is still overeating whichever you look at it. Two examples of healthy foods that are significantly high in calories are seeds and nuts. They contain micronutrients, omega 3 and phytogens that are absolutely wonderful for your health but are excessively high in calories. Don't avoid them; just stick to eating a small handful at a time.

Mistake Number 5 – Your training regime is not intensive enough

While it is important for complete beginners to start off slowly, you should gradually up your game, as you become more and more used to the gym machines, weights and the actual exercise

The key is to relax and, although that is easier said than done, if you can learn some deep breathing, meditation, or yoga and incorporate it every day in your diet, you will see a significant change in your overall health and in your physique

Mistake 8 – You are not sleeping enough

Sleek deprivation also raises cortisol levels and, when you are lacking in sleep; your insulin sensitivity is also reduced. Together, these two problems are not good news for anyone who wants to burn fat. Sleep is a priority in your life. You cannot possibly party all night and expect to function well the next day. Aim for 8 hours of good sleep every single night. Don't drink alcohol, don't use your tablet, mobile phone or watch TV for at least an hour before you go to bed, eliminate caffeine in the evenings and give yourself time to relax in the evenings.

Nicholas Bjorn

Chapter 6 – Eat Right For Weight Loss

From what most of you have read in numerous articles and papers and, of course, the grand old Internet, there are about a gazillion diets to follow. People religiously begin one in the month of January and drop out mid-way due to sheer fatigue, exhaustion, and the primal urge to eat. Almost all diets work in the short term - by eliminating one or more crucial food groups, such as carbs or fat or vegetables or any combination of the groups. That is why, by forcing yourself to eat fewer calories per meal, you definitely lose weight in the beginning. But later on, as your body demands the lost nutrition, you begin bingeing on unhealthy foods and snacks and promptly gain all the weight you managed to lose. That's sad, really. But there's no denying it - you can't fool your body.

But there's a way out. You really don't have to starve or deprive yourself of eating your favorite foods. You can do that and STILL beat the escalating calories. Is it magic? Is it like entering the world of wizards? Is it some alternate realm of reality?

Not really. It's a basic, most fundamental fact of biology. Losing weight happens simply because you consume fewer calories than you burn. That's it. No complicated charts and figures. If you eat less and expend more calories, you lose weight. How this happens is important.

First, we need to understand what a calorie is and what all the fuss is about it.

Simply put, a calorie is a unit of energy. All our foods and drinks give us some kind of energy, the fuel for our body. Carbohydrates, fats, proteins, minerals, and vitamins - all have calories. How much energy they give out is measured by calories. Each day, our body requires a certain number of calories for its normal function - for your heartbeats, brain activity, body functions, etc. So, just in order to EXIST, you expend calories. This is called the Total Daily Energy Expenditure or TDEE. For example, if you are a 40-year-old female, weighing 140 pounds and standing 5"5' tall, you burn 1350 calories by just existing. Similarly, the calorie expenditure of a 30-year-old male, weighing 240 pounds and being 6 feet tall is around 2300. Get a general idea?

Basal Metabolic Rate (BMR)

BMR is basically the number of calories required by your body for its daily function. This base number of calories is required for involuntary functions of the body, such as breathing, pumping of the heart, digestion, etc. According to the Academy of Nutrition and Dietetics, your BMR should not drop below 1200. If it does, it starts affecting your metabolism in a bad way. Muscle mass begins to decrease; body fat falls below acceptable levels, circulation and pulse rate is affected, brain function is affected. Your overall health declines, which is precisely what you DO NOT want.

Factors such as gender, weight, and height affect this number. For a rough estimate, about two-thirds of the calories you eat go into the daily function of your body. The other third portion goes into the motion-related activities of your body. This also depends on the activity levels of your body.

Sedentary Lifestyle: BMR x 1.2

Slightly Active: BMR x 1.375

Moderately Active: BMR x 1.55

Very Active: BMR x 1.725

Now, let us show you an example. You are a 35-year-old male, weighing 200 pounds and standing 72 inches tall (six feet).

Let's use some numbers:

Suppose you're male, 35 years old, weigh 200 pounds and are six feet even (72 inches).

BMR= 1882 calories

If you are a sedentary person, this number jumps to 2258. That means you need that many calories just to sustain yourself on a daily basis, do your tasks, work, etc. If you are a moderately active person, your TDEE comes to 2917.

Now see the difference between being sedentary and moderately active. It amounts to 659 calories. That equals one whole meal! And that is why I wrote in the beginning- we tend to underestimate how much we are eating, but overestimate how much we are expending.

When you eat something, your body has three categories to decide where all those calories will go:

- for fuel-burning
- for rebuilding muscles
- for storing as fat

When you expend as many calories as you consume, you reach something called a "calorie equilibrium." No more, no less. Just a pleasant state of homeostasis. If you want to lose weight, you will need to eat fewer calories. This forces your body to hit the calorie reserve it has to burn fuel.

Now, when you eat more and burn fewer calories, the body does not need the extra calories it just ate. So, they are stored as fat, a.k.a, weight gain. And when you begin to see sense and burn off those extra calories or eat a calorie deficit, you lose weight. Simple?

Sure, in theory. But life isn't this simple, right. We are super amazing at underplaying the amount of food we eat and overestimating the rate at which we burn it off. Human nature, really! The so-called cheat days between exercise regimes, the accidental over-eating of your favorite dessert at a party, or someone's birthday - these are just some of the umpteen excuses we give ourselves when confronted with the reality.

Metabolism and Weight Loss

Your resting metabolism slows down when you lose weight. This is a simple concept. Because there is less of you to fuel and process, your metabolism doesn't have to work that hard to keep your bodily functions intact and functioning properly. When you lose weight, you also lose some water, lean tissue, and fat. If you weigh less, it will have less weight to carry around; the heart will have to pump less, etc. The body will, therefore, burn fewer calories than it did when you carried all that extra weight.

If you look at estimates from a calorie calculator, here's how much the resting calorie burn is for three different weights.

- 2600 calories for 300 lbs
- 2300 calories for 250 lbs
- 2000 calories for 200 lbs.

See the difference? By weighing just 50 pounds less, you strike off 300 calories from your metabolism. But here's where things get interesting. There is something called "adaptive thermogenesis." It basically means that the body keeps adjusting itself to the number of calories consumed and burnt per day, and the process it takes to preserve the body fat within.

Stop Dieting

Our body is constantly wondering if it will get the next meal or not. Because it does that, it has a tendency to store the calories as surplus - just in case the Earth is invaded, and we are left without supplies. That is why even though people seem to lose a few pounds, they have to make a consistent and lifelong effort to keep the extra kilos off. Many other factors - such as environmental changes, psychological elements, medication, depression, emotional pain, anxiety, and other issues can trigger or change eating patterns.

Now, instead of worrying about calories every single time you look at food, it's far, far better to eat the healthy and right kind of foods in the first place. For example - protein (meat, legumes), carbohydrates (brown or white rice, quinoa, wheat), fruit and vegetables, nuts, dairy (if you are not lactose intolerant). Just keep eating these foods and stay happy, full, and healthy for a long, long time. These wholesome foods keep us full for a much longer time, yet aren't that calorie-dense. If you do this over a consistent period of time, you will lose weight.

So, what can you eat to lose weight in a healthy manner?

Protein

As you have learned already, protein is the building block for our skin, hair, and muscles. If eaten properly, it makes for a very filling and delicious food group. Generally speaking, you should eat about 1 gram of protein per lb. of bodyweight. Guzzling a can of energy drink will fill you up for about ten minutes. And leave you with loads of unwanted calories. The same amount of calories can be obtained from a good serving of chicken. Healthier, right? Because protein requires energy to metabolize, a high protein diet can be key for a calorie deficit. It fights the primary cause of weight gain - cravings. Protein can be found in meat, legumes, fowl, eggs, fish, etc. But try to keep the upper limit at 250 grams, because too much of anything can also cause problems.

Vegetables

No, pizza is not a vegetable. Real vegetables are rich in nutrients and calorie-light. That means you can eat a lot of these and feel full but are very unlikely to gain weight. Every meal should have at least two servings of differently colored vegetables - the more color, the better. Seasonal vegetables work best. Broccoli, spinach, cauliflower, radish, Brussels sprouts, kale, zucchini, cucumber, carrots, onions, potatoes, asparagus, etc. are some veggies to get you interested!

Fat

Yes, I said fat. Fat has always been vilified, but healthy fats work wonders for your body and especially for your skin. Foods such as avocado, nuts, olive oil, peanut butter, whole milk, grass-fed butter, etc. contain healthy fat needed by the body. Consume these in small amounts to reap maximum benefits and also lose weight in the process.

The Grain is a Go-Go

Instead of highly processed junk food like pizza, burgers, patties, ready to eat meals and soups, cakes and cookies, go for whole grains. Choose whole-wheat pasta, brown bread, bran, rye crackers, etc. These will fill you up and keep you satiated for a longer time.

Minimize Processed Food

If it's not growing on a tree or swimming in the sea or pulled up from the Earth, don't bother eating it. Processed food is designed to be super tasty but, in reality, contains a whole lot of preservatives and additives. It does make people addicted to it.

Oversee Liquid Calories

Fruit juices and those who say "enriched fruit or energy water" are nothing but sugar in a liquid form. All of your sodas and colas also fall into this category. Liquid calories account for why people can't seem to lose weight even after switching to healthier diets. Even seemingly harmless coffee orders contain lots of cream and sugar. These drinks and beverages have no fiber and only sugar inside them, which wreaks havoc with our bodily systems. Alcohol also does the same - provide empty calories and a hangover which nobody wants. Sugar not only causes obesity but a host of other diseases. If you want your weight loss to work, drink lots of water, black or green tea, or sparkling water. That's it, no sugary beverages.

Drink More Water

This is such an important point; it has been dealt with in another chapter in the book. Drinking water has been found to increase the number of calories you burn. Studies have shown that drinking about eight glasses of water per day is equal to having burnt about 96 extra calories. Sweet deal! Of course, WHEN you drink, it is also important. Drinking water half an hour before meals help reduce hunger, and thus, you eat less, creating a calorie deficit. Also, drinking water half an hour after meals are also beneficial to digestion.

Because the thirst and hunger centers are located so close to each other in the hypothalamus, most of the time, in between meals, we tend to feel hungry when, in fact, we are THIRSTY. Drinking water will curb this pang of false hunger, and you will eat properly when the actual mealtime comes around.

Condiments and Accompaniments

If your healthy broccoli, pear and carrot salad has a generous overdose of ketchup and mayo over it, or if you dunk everything in heavy sauces and dips, the actual nutritional value becomes less. Keep an eye on what you put on your veggies and meats.

Smaller Meals

Food nutrition experts also recommend that you eat smaller meals and pace them throughout the day. This keeps your blood sugar levels in check and also stops you from overindulging on unhealthy snacks.

Smart Substitutions

Don't want to eat salad by itself? Add some vinegar, soy sauce, and basil for an instant livening up of the situation. Homemade salsa and hummus, mustard paste, homemade white butter for your jacket potatoes, basil and cilantro, lemon, and vinegar are all healthy complements and dressings for your pasta, salad, and toppings.

What Else Can I Do?

Predetermine your Meals

I know it sounds like a boring and tedious activity. But picture this - you're home tired after a long day's work, and maybe managed to squeeze in some exercise in between. But you're too tired to cook, so you just order some pizza and a soda, and all your hard work go down the drain. Pre-plan and pre-cook your meals and bung them in the freezer. It makes a world of difference in your weight loss journey.

Strength Train

I can't stress this enough. When you lift weights, you force your muscles to break down. And when you rest and eat properly, the muscles rebuild themselves and take the fuel from the stores available in your body. That means, even as you are resting, you are burning calories. It's a win-win all the way - as you keep getting stronger, your muscles become bigger, and you keep losing body fat. This is also an important aspect of losing weight and maintaining it and is discussed in a separate chapter.

Calorie Deficit

Consistently maintain a calorie deficit. You can also mix and match your exercise routines to include cardio, strength training, Zumba, Pilates, yoga, etc. and continue with your healthy weight loss journey.

Step Up!

Even if you can't find the time to strength train, you can always start walking. That remains the best and most natural exercise ever designed for the body. Move constantly. Park your car a few hundred yards from your office or home. Take the stairs at work. Walk back from the supermarket. Run around with your dog or your neighbor's dog. March in place while watching advertisements. Just keep moving it.

Close your Kitchen at Night

Late-night snacking in front of the TV, eating because you don't have anything else to do or simply dipping your hand inside the cookie jar every time you enter the kitchen - these are just some of the ways in which you pile on unnecessary pounds. Set a time for your meals and stick to it. Get into the habit of closing up the kitchen after a set time, say 9 p.m. No going into the kitchen or fridge after that. If it helps, brush your teeth an hour after eating. The minty taste will let you forget any mindless snacking you might want to indulge in.

Controlling your Immediate Environment

If your fridge is always stocked with pastries, cakes, sodas, pizzas, and the like, it's very unlikely that you will reach for a bag of cauliflower or carrots when there is an appetizing cheese burst pizza staring at you. Make it a point to stock your pantry and fridge with healthy foods - vegetables, fruit, healthy cuts of meat, nuts, olive oil, whole grains, popcorn, lemon water, etc. so that when you feel the urge to snack or make yourself a meal, you reach out for real food.

One Step at a Time

I get it. You're ambitious and want to lose ten pounds by this Saturday. But if you cut back on your favorite foods, begin a vigorous strength training regime, say bye-bye to alcohol and keep moving all the time - you will most definitely hit a plateau very soon. Take it slowly. Cut back on one unhealthy snack per week. Or have one glass of wine in two weeks. Go for a walk first instead of lifting weights straight away. Take it slowly and steadily.

Check Food Labels

Whenever buying something from the market, be sure to check the nutrition label on the back. If it lists more than ten chemicals and just one or two real food names, chuck it back on the shelf. It's not worth eating it. For example - potato chips should be just that; Potatoes, oil, and salt rather than some twenty triglycerides and ten preservatives shown on the label.

Forgive Yourself

If you ate unhealthy food at one meal, it's okay. It's not the end of the world. Get back on track with your next meal.

You can use some popular apps to keep track of how many calories you are consuming. My Fitness Pal, Fat Secret, and Lose It are three of the most popular ones right now.

Of course, you can't be tracking your food for the rest of your life. But, when you're starting out, it helps to know how much you are eating. That will help you see if you are going overboard with some food groups or ignoring something else completely. Portion sizes also matter here. Let's show you an example.

One pound of fat is equal to something like 3500 calories. So, if you wish to lose one pound of fat per week, you need to eat 500 calories less per day. You can do that either by cutting out 500 calories or burning them through exercise. And arguably, it is much more difficult to increase time for activity levels than it is to reduce calorie consumption. Let's face it - if given a choice, which would you pick? Incorporating thirty minutes or more of exercise time in your schedule or giving up and substituting a food group in your diet?

You guessed it.

Let's take 200 calories as a measure. 200 calories of broccoli would fill up a dinner plate. The same 200 calories are found in half a Snickers bar. How many people you know would prefer eating broccoli to a bar of chocolate? And is it easier to eat a full plate of broccoli than a tempting half bar of yummy chocolate? And who the heck ever eats HALF a bar of chocolate?

That is why you need to eat REAL foods.

Chapter 7 – Planning Your Meals

Meal planning may seem to be quite a difficult task, but it really isn't. It is easy and doable if you know and understands what you are doing. In simple terms, meal planning means planning your meals for the week and keeping things ready for these meals. This way, you can save a lot of time and money. Meal planning can be divided into three sections:

- Select the recipes

- Shop for the ingredients

- Prepare the ingredients

Many people find meal planning difficult because many myths that are prevalent about it. For instance, a lot of people believe that you need to plan meals by noting them down in huge binders, which you need to lug around all the time. But this is false; you can make simple meals in Google Docs or any notepad application on your phone. If you do not like using your phone for lists, you can also make simple lists on paper and post it on your fridge.

Many people also think that meal planning is only suitable for large families. But this is false. You can make meal plans for yourself as well. This is especially recommended if you are trying to lose weight or are an extremely busy person. It is also recommended for people who are trying to save money.

Meal planning does not take a lot of work, especially if you have the basics ready. Once you have the basics ready, you can make meal plans for every week in less than an hour.

Meal plans are extremely flexible, and you can change and experiment according to your needs and desires. Nothing is set in stone in the world of meal plans.

Beginning a Meal Plan

Before making a plan, you need to ask yourself:

Why do I need a meal plan?

There are no wrong answers to the above question, but focusing on the reason will allow you to concentrate effectively. In the beginning, keep your reasons and meal plans simple. You can increase the difficulty level with time and experience.

Once you have understood your reason behind meal planning, you can now start with the plan itself. As said above, the first step for meal planning is choosing recipes.

Choosing Recipes

Choosing recipes is a simple task if you know the reason behind your meal plan. For instance, if you are making meal plans because you want to lose weight, it is recommended to choose only healthy recipes. Similarly, if you are making meal plans because you are trying to cut down your expenses, then you should choose recipes that do not require a lot of exotic or expensive ingredients. Thus, you need to focus on the reason behind your meal plan all the time. Never choose recipes randomly. Similarly, avoid making meal plans a day before (at least in the beginning.) Give yourself at least three days to make a meal plan and prepare for it.

If you eat out frequently, add these outings to your meal plan. Once you decide the days and meals, you can move on to the recipes. It is recommended to choose recipes according to your schedule. For instance, if you are generally the busiest on Thursdays, you can either opt for a simple recipe, or you can opt for a recipe that can be made in a slow cooker. This way, you can just add the ingredients to the cooker in the morning and let it cook over low temperature until you return. If you work late on Mondays, you can make more food on Sunday and carry it the next day.

Once you have noted down the recipes, it is now time to get the ingredients.

Ingredients

To make the shopping easy, it is recommended to make two-ingredient lists- a master list and a grocery list. Two lists may sound to be a lot more work than one single list, but making a master list will help you a lot in the long term. The master list will help you keep a stock of fresh and dried ingredients in your pantry, and you won't have to buy them every week.

Master List

In this, add the ingredients that are used in almost all the recipes. You can also add ingredients that are generally purchased in bulk on this list. Try to avoid easily perishable ingredients to this list.

Grocery List

In this list, add anything that can be stored for at least a couple of days. This should include vegetables, dairy, eggs, etc.

Once you have collected the ingredients, the next step in meal planning is preparing them.

Keeping your ingredients prepared is a great way to save time and money. Keeping things prepared is especially great for people who want to avoid working on weekends. Keeping things prepared can help you avoid frustration and fatigue. It will allow you to have more free time for yourself. It is recommended to set aside a few hours on Sunday (or any other day that you are free) and prepare your ingredients according to your meal plan. For instance, if you plan to make salads on Monday or Tuesday, it is recommended to chop some things and refrigerate them. Similarly, if you plan to make pasta or any similar product, you can keep the ingredients for the sauce, such as garlic, etc. ready. Keeping things clean can also save you a lot of time.

Meal plans are simple and effective if you know how to craft them and follow them successfully.

Chapter 8 – The Importance of Water

Water, water everywhere; all the boards did shrink,

Water, water everywhere, nor any drop to drink

The Rime of the Ancient Mariner

Water is everywhere around us, isn't it? That gorgeous pool, those tantalizing lakes and ponds, those mighty seas and majestic oceans of the planet. Over 80 percent of the planet is basically water. And it's the same case with our bodies too. Water makes up a whopping 65 to 70 percent of our bodies. Two atoms of hydrogen, one of oxygen. And it powers the planet. It's not only vital for life to survive and thrive. Going without it for as little as three days will send you into an irreversible spiral of decline.

Now, why is this compound so essential to our health?

Water performs some of the most important functions of the human body: flushing out waste products, regulating body temperature, keeping homeostasis going on properly, aiding brain functions, and more.

Benefits of Drinking Water

Creation of Saliva

Do you know how dry and irritable the mouth gets when you have a fever or some other disease that dries up your mouth? You miss your saliva terribly during those times. Saliva is nothing but water, mucus, and enzymes that break down your food and keep your mouth healthy and germ-free. If you drink water regularly, your body produces enough saliva for proper function. A dry mouth usually indicates dehydration.

Regulation of Body Temperature

Every time you breathe or blink, you lose water through the pores of your skin and eyes. Hydration of the body is vital for the proper regulation of your body temperature. You lose more water through sweat when you exercise or live in hot environments. Sweating keeps your body cool, but the temperature will rise if the loss of water is not replenished. So, keep drinking water to keep your basal metabolic temperature right.

Protection of Tissues, Joints, and Spinal Cord

Water acts as a lubricant and cushions your bones and joints from everyday jarring and bumping around. It eases their function.

Waste Removal

Water is like a carrier of waste material outside your body. By way of sweating, urination, and defecation, water helps flush out toxic waste from your body. Not doing so will result in painful constipation, kidney problems, kidney stones, metabolic breakdown, and a slow build-up of toxins in the body. A build-up of waste in the body can result in bloating and gas in the stomach. People may also feel very lethargic. Generous doses of water throughout the day can help curb this problem.

Maximize Physical Activities and Exertions

During physical activity, a lot of water is lost due to perspiration. Athletes may lose up to 6 to 10 percent of body weight during rigorous training. Drinking plenty of water during such activities helps keep the body cool and energized. Not being hydrated affects your strength and stamina for sports and physical activity. If you exercise in the heat, without drinking adequate water, you may be in danger of serious medical maladies such as heat stroke, hyperthermia, low blood pressure, etc.

Prevention of Constipation

Fiber is a must to have smooth and easy bowel movements. But water aids immensely in the process too. If you don't drink water throughout the day, you might have constipation. The only way out is to drink a couple of glasses of water, wait for an hour or so and then go to the restroom. You will find that the bowel movement is now significantly easier.

Aids in Digestion

Drinking water half an hour before and after meals has been proven to have a positive effect on weight loss and digestion. When you have it before eating, you feel less hungry and eat less. When you drink water half an hour after meals, it won't interfere with the natural digestive processes and helps churn the food easily.

Nutrient Absorption

Water also helps your body to absorb nutrients, vitamins, minerals from food, and delivers these important components to the rest of the body for its building and strengthening activities.

Weight Loss

There are numerous studies linking weight loss and water consumption. While dieting or exercising or just eating healthy, drinking water in adequate amounts also amounts to losing extra pounds.

Fights off Illnesses

Drinking enough water is a natural remedy to ward off diseases like kidney stones, urinary tract infections, hypertension, etc. Water is also a carrier of essential nutrients and vitamins throughout the body, so whatever you eat will be distributed well.

Boosts Energy

Metabolism is also affected by water or lack of it. Drinking water activates the metabolic levels, which, in turn, boosts the energy levels. Studies have shown that as little as 500 ml. of water can increase the metabolism by about 30 percent.

Mood Enhancer

I'm sure you've had bad days, or know of people who became grumpy for no reason at all. Dehydration is also a cause of these kinds of mood swings. It results in fatigue, anxiety, and grumpiness. A bit of water will do the trick!

Skin Lover

We all know the benefits of water for our skin. As the water flushes out toxins from the body, the water which goes into our cells plumps them up. This, in turn, plumps up the skin cells and surfaces and also promotes collagen production, resulting in fewer wrinkles and a more youthful you!

Prevention of Overall Dehydration

We all know how dangerous dehydration is. Severe dehydration can result in kidney failure, brain swelling, seizure, and other body dysfunction. Water helps prevent all these situations. Keep drinking enough water at intervals to sustain a healthy body.

How Much Water Should I Drink?

According to the National Academies of Sciences, Engineering, and Medicine, these are the guidelines for water intake for most people:

Around 125 ounces each day for men and 93 ounces for women. Of course, it all varies depending on the type of work one does and the environment one lives in. Food gives us about 20 percent of our daily intake of water. Everything else depends on how much water and how many water-based drinks you ingest throughout the day.

The color of your urine and thirst you experience are also indicators of your hydration levels. Pale yellow-colored urine is a good indication, while dark yellow means you need to drink more water.

Keep a bottle of water with you and drink from it at regular intervals. As a rule of thumb, aim to drink at least three to four liters of water in a day. Of course, if you end up drinking too much water, that will cause irreparable damage to your body and brain. Just drink enough to sustain and maintain good metabolism.

Water and its Many Forms

Water is just that, right? Plain old boring water? But what about juices, sodas, smoothies, colas, sugary teas, etc.? Sure, they are hydrating and feel particularly great on a hot day, but they also contain enormous quantities of sugar and unwanted calories. Coffee and tea are diuretics - they make you lose water. Alcohol also gives the impression of being hydrating, but it actually has the opposite effect. The same goes for sports drinks. Though they contain electrolytes and other energy-giving substances, they also contain sugar and salt, which is more than the recommended amount. Pay attention to the number of such drinks when you do consume them.

The Role of Water in Weight Loss

Many studies have highlighted the correlation between drinking water and weight loss. Let us see how it does that:

Burns More Calories

When you drink more water, it increases the number of calories burnt by the body, also known as the "resting energy expenditure" of the body. Some studies have shown that within 10 minutes of drinking water, the energy expenditure increases by about 30 percent! And this effect lasts for a whole hour. Another study conducted among overweight women showed that drinking just one liter of water extra per day resulted in a loss of almost 2 kilos over a period of a year. There were no other control variables here - no exercise or lifestyle changes. Just the additional drinking of one liter of water. Therefore, the results are really impressive. Also, the study revealed that just half an extra liter of water per day would cause you to burn 23 calories. This results in a massive 17,000 calorie burn over the whole year!

Natural Appetite Suppressant

We have spoken about the hunger and thirst centers located in the hypothalamus, in a different section of this book. When the stomach senses that its capacity is now full, it sends a signal to the hypothalamus, which in turn gives a feeling of "fullness" to the eater. Drinking water before meals can fool the brain into thinking that it is somewhat full, thus avoiding overeating. Because those two centers are so closely located, a person may think he or she is hungry, when thirst might be the actual issue. Drinking water also curbs unnecessary snacking between healthy meals.

Curbs Unwanted Liquid Calorie Intake

Sodas, colas, sugary drinks, fruit juices, etc. contain a large amount of sugar, which needlessly build-up problems in the body. Drinking water at regular intervals ensures that one doesn't fall prey to such liquid calories.

A Friend to Fat Burning

Water is essential to help burn fat. Without adequate water in the body, the process of metabolizing fat, called "lipolysis," cannot occur properly. The first step, called "hydrolysis," happens only in the presence of water - where the water molecules interact with triglycerides for the creation of glycerol and fatty acids. You have to drink enough water to keep this process going on smoothly and to burn fat effectively.

Workout Helper

Eating healthy and exercises are two sides of the same coin. And water helps immensely with exercise and workouts. It lubricates the joints, muscles, and tendons effectively and makes them more pliable for exercise, thus helping you on your way toward a healthy and happy body.

Chapter 9 – Strength Training: A Vital Component of Your Weight Loss Journey

When you exercise and pick something you love to do, you give the best workout to your body and mind. You are also motivated further to keep eating healthy and keep moving.

Don't feel like exercising? It must be something you LOVE to do. Don't do it because your neighbor/friend/dad told you to. If you hate running or gymming or Pilates, don't do it! Pick something you love and stick to it.

Remember, you read somewhere in this book that whatever you eat is taken inside by the body for three functions: fuel, storing as fat, and rebuilding muscles, when you weight train and challenge your muscles beyond their capacity, the body's sorting behavior changes.

There's really nothing like lightweight training, so we'll leave that. A heavy workout would include a 500 lb. deadlift or 450 lb. squats. Intense bodyweight training for strength might include a handstand push up or 100 pull-ups in a minute. You get the drift.

Now when you weight train - you pick something heavy and move it against gravity for a certain number of times - your muscles break down. When you rest, eat, and sleep, they rebuild themselves in the next 48 hours. So, talking about the redirecting of calories, which happens, the body sends those calories to rebuild the broken down muscles. Also, it will direct the additional calories to burn as fuel to handle all this intense lifting activity.

So what does that mean for metabolism and weight loss? Metabolism gets a boost, and you burn calories even as you are

Chapter 10 – Kitchen Implements and Gadgets for Healthy Cooking

Now that you are truly on your way to eating and living healthy, why not arm yourself with the right kind of tools and gadgets which will help you stick to your health plan? Here's a handy list of implements to have in your kitchen.

Steamer

Steam your vegetables for salads and veggie bowls easily.

Handheld Spiralizer

No more buying noodles and pasta from the take-out! Just use this handy spiralizer to carve your own noodles and pasta shapes at home.

Blender

A godsend for kitchens. Blend your fruit and nuts into smoothies, whip up healthy juices, and just about any dip or sauce that you like. All at the press of a button!

Nonstick Grill

This can be electric or the one you set on the stove. Grill your meats and sandwiches to perfection with the nonstick grill.

Some even come with a charcoal flavor, to give you that barbeque feeling.

Rice Cooker

Another life-saving device. You can bung in your rice, measure out the water, and turn it on. By the time you're done with other activities, your rice is also done. Simply take it out and have it with whatever meats or veggies you cooked.

Nonstick Frying Pan

Takes up less oil, and you also get your meats and veggies out of it cleanly and easily.

Handheld Immersion Blender

This is different from the regular blender. With this, you plunge the blender into the foods you wish to blend. Making buttermilk, squashes, and other quick mixing drinks has never been easier!

Vegetable Peeler cum Julienne

This gadget allows you to do two things. Julienne, or cut vegetables into thin, long sticks and also peel tough veggies such as carrots and gourds.

Measuring Cups

Of course, at some point, you will want to bake and cook like a pro. These measuring cups come in very handy, having all kinds of metric conversions and quantities written clearly.

Tupperware and Prep Containers

After having worked all that hard to cook, you may have leftovers. Keep them fresh and safe inside Tupperware containers, which are microwave and dishwasher safe.

Food Processor

If you can afford this, congratulations. You've saved yourself precious hours in the kitchen. A food processor will do all these for you - chopping, dicing, slicing, shredding, mincing, pureeing, and even mixing batters and doughs! A small kitchen miracle in itself.

Nicholas Bjorn

Chapter 11 – Refrigerator Essentials for Healthy Eating

When you are surrounded by packets of chips, cans of soda, bags of pretzels, or boxes of pizza, it's really hard to even begin thinking healthily. Why not stock up your larder and refrigerator with something healthy, so that whenever you feel hungry and reach out, you will always hit something which is real food - not junk food.

Here are some foods and condiments you can keep in your fridge/pantry/freezer for continuing your healthy streak:

1. Basic Vegetables: You can store veggies like carrots, beans, celery, bell peppers, eggplant, etc. because they can stay for at least a week or so in the fridge. Just put them inside mesh bags so they can breathe properly.

2. Fruit: Apples, pears, grapes, melons, berries, citrus fruits can be stored for a good amount of time in the fridge. These make for a very healthy and tasty snack too.

3. Greens: The thing with greens is that they begin to wilt and spoil easily. So, keep your greens like kale, spinach, cilantro, and lettuce in large mesh bags or containers with drainboards underneath them. Keep them this way for a week at most.

4. Herbs: The top choices for herbs are cilantro, thyme, parsley, sage, rosemary, and dill. These can be stored fresh or in the dried form. If fresh, wrap them in dry paper and store.

5. Dried fruit: Another quick snack is dried fruit and nuts. You can store almonds, cashews, peanuts, cranberries, blueberries, dried figs, apricots, and raisins for a really long time. Use them in baking and cooking and enjoy the delicious taste. A small handful of nuts is enough to fill you up for a long time.

6. Milk: Keep a variety of milk such as almond, cashew, soy, rice, or hemp milk easily available at markets. Use them in breakfast cereal, baking, or cooking. But yes, have them sparingly.

7. Eggs: One of nature's best and cheapest nutritional hacks. When you're hungry, just boil a couple of eggs and have them with some salt and pepper. Or, scramble some eggs with butter and seasonings and have it on top of whole-wheat toast. The possibilities with eggs are limitless and equally healthy.

8. Salsa: You can either make your own salsa or buy a jar from the market. It is a delicious dip, dressing, and sauce - or simply have it with some baked sweet potato fries.

9. Mustard: Another delicious fall back option for sandwiches, stir-fries, sauces, and dressings.

10. Yeast: Store this in the active or dry form. Yeast adds a cheesy flavor to foods and is used in baking - for bread and pizza bases. Try some in your pasta and savory dishes as well.

11. Miso paste: This is a mild yet rich flavoring agent. Try it with your sauces and dips.

12. Tahini/ Nut butter: A super delicious and healthy snack would be nut butter with some crackers. Peanut and

almond butter are especially suitable for this purpose, and can also be used with sandwiches and baked stuff.

13. Soy sauce: Mostly used in Chinese cooking along with vinegar and chili sauces, you can also use soy sauce as a dressing or in salads or just one spoonful of it in a sauce - to embrace its taste and goodness.

14. Cacao powder: A fat-free and super yummy baking essential, keep some handy in your pantry or fridge to quickly whip up delicious low-calorie desserts.

For Your Freezer

1. Cooked beans: Suppose you made an extra helping of beans. Save time for the next meal by simply freezing this portion. To reuse, thaw the bag out in the fridge overnight, or run hot water over them and consume.

2. Cooked grains: Because grains take a long time to cook, it makes sense to make a larger quantity and freeze the leftovers. Storing cooked grains like rice and quinoa in the freezer will make the next meal planning a breeze.

3. Frozen vegetables: Frozen veggies such as corn, peas, carrots, cauliflower, edamame, etc. will ensure that you always have a healthy meal option to fall back on, instead of relying on take-outs.

4. Frozen fruit: Whenever there is a grocery sale, stock up on basic fruit like berries, apples, bananas, lemons, cantaloupes, grapefruit, etc. Again, a time-saving meal option.

5. Ginger and garlic: These are basic seasoning herbs and freeze very well too. Just grind together equal quantities of ginger and garlic, fry them in a little oil and when cool, put in freezer bags and freeze. Whenever you want to make a meat or veggie-based dish, just put together your frozen veggies, take the herbs from the fridge and cook them with some pre-roasted ginger and garlic and you have a meal ready in no time!

6. Corn, Rice, and Wheat Tortillas: You can quickly make wraps, tacos, and quesadillas if you have a ready store of these items in your freezer.

Chapter 12 – How to Eat Healthy Without Going Broke and Losing Your Mind

Now, eating healthy and all is great. But if you're a college student or someone who is on a tight budget or similar, it's more tempting to give in to a cheap bagel or pizza at the diner than laboriously check grocery prices and lug home bags of produce and herbs. It is even easier to just pop in a bag full of Doritos rather than get up earlier in the mornings to pack your lunch.

Yep, I hear you. But, it turns out, there are easy hacks everywhere. You can begin your healthiness quotient right now.

Love coffee and can't give it up? Cut back just one cup a day. Or bring in some homemade coffee in a flask. Another better option is to switch to green tea. Leave your tea leaves at work and bring along a hot water brewer. There is really no downside to deciding to start eating healthy. The thing is- when your body keeps getting empty calories by way of unhealthy snacks, it assumes that it will go on forever. When you suddenly start feeding it healthy stuff, it will rebel for a few days, then quickly adjust. The cravings slowly disappear, and the body starts demanding and utilizing healthy food you put into it. All this will result in a happy and sound you!

Shopping the Right Way for Health

Frequent One or Two Stores

Of course, keep an eye out on different offers, but frequent one or two places where you've been before. Check what is on sale and pick the best foods in that. Meats, veggies, fruit- doesn't matter. Pick out the best and freshest produce on display, not necessarily based on the menu you have planned for the week. Bring everything home, and THEN plan your menus. It will save you a lot of time and money.

Get Creative while Cooking

Let's say a recipe calls for green peppers, but you have yellow ones. Or it says hummus, and you forgot to buy chickpeas. There are always substitutions available. Check your pantry and fridge. Use yellow bell peppers instead of green. Or, use some miso dip instead of hummus.

Prepare Meals in Advance

It's quite easy to do this. You can chop your veggies and make batters or doughs while binge-watching your favorite shows. Even better, you can cook your chicken and veggies, portion them out and freeze them in individual serving boxes. That way, you just have to bung one in the oven before you come to work and won't have to depend on any store-bought food item for your lunch.

Buy in Bulk

Whenever possible, look out for bargains in meats and produce. Buy a whole bunch of it when on sale or discount, chop them into meal-sized portions and either freeze them immediately or cook them and then freeze.

Eat Small and Healthy Snacks

Stuff like fruit, peanut butter on crackers, carrot sticks, sprouts, popcorn, nuts are all healthy and filling snack options if you get hungry in between meals.

Eat Everything You Buy

More often than not, we go out in a rush and buy tons of food and produce and stash it all in the fridge. After about a week of hard work cooking and making meals, we fall off the wagon, and all that food keeps rotting inside the fridge. That's such a waste of money. Make it a point to stock only about a week's worth of produce and meats in your fridge and EAT ALL OF IT before you buy new food.

Learn to Cook

It doesn't necessarily have to be a Michelin rated meal. Even something as simple as scrambled eggs on toast, chicken breasts marinated and grilled, healthy low-fat sandwiches or rice wraps filled with vegetables are all great and simple starting points for meals. Pick one simple recipe and master it. Then another, and another. You can definitely learn to cook elaborate and complicated meals later on, but for now, this will do.

Nicholas Bjorn

Chapter 13 – 15 Tasty Super Food Smoothies Recipes

The following recipes all contain superfoods and are another alternative as a way of making sure that you get all you need in your diet. With the smoothies, simply add all the ingredients to your blender, whiz them up and enjoy!

Peanut Butter Power Shake

- 1 scoop of whey protein powder, chocolate flavored
- 1 tbsp. organic or natural peanut butter
- ½ banana
- 1 cup of almond milk
- Ice cubes

Dark Chocolate Shake

- 1 scoop whey protein , chocolate flavored
- 1 cup almond milk
- 2 ½ tbsp. cacao powder
- 2 ice cubes

Anti-Aging Kiwi-Blueberry Smoothie

- 1/2 scoop whey protein, vanilla
- 1/2 cup 0% plain Greek yogurt
- 1 cup flax milk
- 2 kiwi
- 1/2 cup blueberries
- 2 ice cubes

Berry Banana Smoothie

- 1 scoop whey protein, vanilla
- 1 cup flax milk
- 1/2 cup blackberries
- 1/2 banana
- 1/2 cup raspberries
- 1/2 cup strawberries
- 2 ice cubes

Peach-Mango Yogurt Smoothie
- 1 Cup plain 0% Greek yogurt
- 1 peach
- 1 cup mango chunks
- 1/4 tsp. cinnamon
- 1 cup ice

The Lean Muscle Mochaccino
- 1 scoop whey protein, mocha cappuccino
- 1.5 cups flax milk
- 2.5 tbsp. cacao powder
- 2 ice cubes

Orange Creamsicle Smoothie
- 1 scoop whey protein, orange creamsicle
- 1 medium orange
- 1 cup almond milk
- 1/2 cup orange juice
- 1 cup water/ice

Liquid Breakfast Smoothie

- 3/4 cup plain 0% Greek yogurt
- 1/2 banana
- 1/4 cup rolled oats
- 1 cup strawberries
- 1 cup water/Ice

Banana Nut Shake

- 1 scoop vanilla whey protein
- 1 cup almond milk
- 1 large banana
- 3 tbsp. organic peanut butter
- water/ice

Strawberry Shortcake Smoothie

- 3/4 cup plain 0% Greek yogurt
- 1 cup strawberries
- 1/2 cup rolled oats
- 1 tsp vanilla extract
- water/ice

Mango Pineapple Shake

- 1 scoop vanilla whey protein
- 1/2 cup mango chunks
- 1/2 cup pineapple chunks
- 1 cup almond Milk

Creamy Chocolate Avocado Smoothie

- 1 scoop chocolate whey protein
- 1/2 small avocado
- 3/4 banana
- 1 1/2 cup ice/Water

Chapter 14 – 5 Tasty Super Food Soup Recipes

Green Superfood Soup

Ingredients:

- 185 g broccoli
- 2 leeks sliced
- 1 onion roughly diced
- ½ teaspoon garlic oil or minced garlic
- 1 cup green split peas – soaked for 1 hour, rinsed
- 310 g medium cauliflower
- 9-10 g dry wakame seaweed – soaked for 10 min, roughly chopped
- 80 g kale – roughly chopped
- ½ cup stock
- pinch sea salt
- pepper
- ¼ tsp thyme
- enough water to cover
- Oil for cooking

- Coconut cream

Instructions:

1. Heat up the oil in a large pan
2. Cook the onions and leeks until they are brown
3. Add all other ingredients, add the stock and enough water to cover the vegetables
4. Simmer for about 1 hour over a low heat, or until the split peas are soft
5. Blend in the blender to make a thick soup
6. Add in some coconut cream and water to bring it to the consistency you like
7. Season with salt and pepper

Carrot and Turmeric Soup

Ingredients:

- 500 g carrots
- 2 garlic cloves
- 1 onion, white
- 1 tbsp. coconut oil
- 2 tsp turmeric
- 1 tbsp. fresh ginger
- 400 ml stock
- 150 ml water
- Salt and pepper
- 1 lime

Instructions:

1. Chop the carrots into pieces about an inch in size and peel the garlic; set aside
2. Cut the onion into small bits and fry over a medium heat with a pinch of salt and 1 tbsp. oil
3. Add the ginger and turmeric and cook for 30 seconds, stirring
4. Crush the garlic and add it in, stir and add the carrots
5. Roast for a few minutes before adding the stock

6. Use a blender to blend the soup until smooth – add more water if needed

7. Add another inch of salt, pepper and squeeze the juice in from the lime

Dairy-Free Creamy Avocado Soup

Ingredients:

- 3 ripe avocado, peeled, pitted and chopped
- 2 cups plain dairy-free yogurt
- ⅓ cup cashews
- ⅓ cup finely chopped fresh cilantro
- ⅓ cup Vidalia onion, chopped
- 1 Tbsp. white balsamic vinegar
- 1 cup green tea, brewed and chilled
- 1 tsp. sea salt
- ¼ tsp. freshly ground white pepper
- 2 chives, finely chopped

Instructions:

1. Blend the avocado, yoghurt, cilantro, almonds, onion, vinegar, green tea, pepper and sea salt until smooth
2. Transfer into a bowl and cover; refrigerate for 2 hours
3. Serve chilled and garnished with chopped chives

Nicholas Bjorn

Spicy Chicken and Quinoa Soup

Ingredients:

- 2 tbsp. extra virgin olive oil
- 1 cup diced onion
- 2 garlic cloves, chopped
- 2 tomatoes, peeled and diced
- 2 carrots, peeled and chopped
- 1 tsp of paprika
- 2 tsp of cumin
- 2 cups of white meat from 2 baked skinless and shredded organic chicken breasts
- 2 cups of filtered water
- 4 cups low sodium organic chicken broth
- 2 cups of fresh or frozen peas
- 2 cups cooked quinoa
- 4 tbsp. finely chopped parsley
- 3 tbsp. finely chopped cilantro
- 1 tsp kosher salt
- Freshly ground black pepper

Instructions:

1. Heat up the olive oil in a large soup pot
2. Add the onions, garlic and sauté until translucent, about 5 minutes
3. Add the tomato, carrots, cumin and pepper, cook for a father 5 minutes, stirring
4. Add the water and broth, turn the heat up to high and bring to a boil
5. Add the peas, quinoa, herbs and chicken, season with salt and peeper
6. Reduce heat and simmer for 25 minutes
7. Serve hot with a diced avocado

To Bake Chicken Breasts

1. Preheat the oven to 350° F
2. Rub olive oil over the chicken and season with salt and pepper
3. Place in a foil lined baking sheet, skin side up and bake for 40 to 45 minutes
4. Remove and allow it to cool off before taking the skin off and shredding it

Nicholas Bjorn

Slow Cooker Superfood Soup

Ingredients:

- 2 cups sliced carrots
- 1 large sweet potato, cut into 1/2" cubes
- 1 cup fresh or frozen green beans
- 1/2 cup fresh cilantro, chopped
- 1 small onion, diced
- 1 clove garlic, minced
- 2 (15 ounce) cans black beans, drained and rinsed
- 1/2 teaspoon crushed red pepper flakes
- 1/2 teaspoon black pepper
- 1 teaspoon chili powder
- 1 teaspoon cumin
- Kosher or sea salt to taste
- 2 cups vegetable juice (I used R.W. Knudsen, Organic Very Veggie Juice, no sugar added)
- 2 cups vegetable broth, low-sodium

Instructions:

1. Mix all the ingredients together in your slow cooker, cover and cook it for about 6-8 hours on low, or until the vegetables have gone tender. If you want, you can add in a tbsp. of low fat cheddar cheese

You can sauté onion in 1 tbsp. olive oil for 5 minutes and then add the garlic and sauté for a further 1 minute before adding them to the slow cooker. You can also add in 2 cups of coarsely chopped kale about 5 minutes before the end of cooking

Chapter 15 – 6 Yummy and Healthy One-Bowl Meals

Quinoa and Chicken Burrito Bowl with Green Sauce

Ingredients:

For the quinoa:

- 1.5 cups pre-washed quinoa
- ¾ tsp salt

For the chicken:

- 2 pounds chicken tenderloin or boneless chicken pounded to ½ inch thickness
- 5 tbsp. extra virgin olive oil
- 2 tsp honey
- 4 garlic cloves, minced
- ½ tsp ground black pepper
- 1 tbsp. lime zest (from two limes)
- 1-1/4 tsp chili powder

- ½ tsp coriander (fresh or dry)
- ¼ tsp dried oregano
- Salt: As per taste

For the green sauce:

- 1 jalapeno chili pepper, seeded and chopped
- 1 cup cilantro leaves
- 2 garlic cloves, chopped
- ¼ cup sour cream
- ½ cup mayonnaise
- 1 tbsp. fresh lime juice
- 2 tbsp. extra virgin olive oil
- Salt and pepper - As per taste

Instructions:

The Chicken

1. Mix all the ingredients except the chicken breasts in a large freezer bag. Close it and thoroughly mix all the ingredients together.
2. Add the chicken breasts into the marinade and mix until every piece is evenly coated with it. Seal the bag and put it

inside the fridge (preferably in a bowl) and let it marinate for at least 6 hours or overnight.

3. When it is fully marinated, take the bag out of the fridge.

4. Clean your grill and put it onto preheat. Spray it with a nonstick cooking spray or lightly coat the grill with oil until it is well oiled.

5. Take the chicken pieces out and lay them on the grill. Slowly grill them for two or three minutes on each side and transfer to a plate. Cut them into bite-sized pieces.

The Quinoa

1. Mix the quinoa, salt, and around two and a half cups of water in a saucepan.

2. Let it come to a boil, then reduce the flame and cover.

3. Cook for ten to fifteen minutes until the quinoa absorbs water and gets cooked. When done, take it out in a bowl and keep aside.

The Sauce

1. Mix all the sauce ingredients in a blender and combine to make a smooth puree. Taste and check for seasonings. If you wish to make it in advance, you can put this sauce into a bowl and refrigerate it until you want to eat.

How to Assemble

Get your quinoa bowl in front of you. Put the grilled chicken on top, and pour the sauce over it. If you wish, you can add additional toppings like tomatoes, diced pumpkin, carrots, or celery.

French Lentil Salad with Goat Cheese

Ingredients:

- 1 cup French lentils (or any other lentils)
- 3 ounces goat cheese
- 3 cups chicken broth
- 1 large carrot, finely chopped
- 2 celery stalks, finely chopped
- 1 small bay leaf
- 1 tsp fresh thyme
- 3 tbsp. parsley, chopped
- 2 garlic cloves, chopped
- 1 tsp mustard
- 1 tsp honey
- Salt: As per taste

Instructions:

1. Wash and rinse the lentils well.

2. Mix lentils, chicken broth, and bay leaf in a saucepan. Let it boil for a few minutes, then simmer them over low heat until the lentils are soft and tender. This may take about 20 to 25 minutes.

3. After this, remove the bay leaf and drain the water from the lentils.

4. In a bowl, mix together all ingredients except the goat cheese.

5. When the lentils are cool, add them to the bowl, adjust seasonings and toss to combine well.

6. Just before eating, crumble the goat cheese over the salad and serve. You may wish to serve the salad with fresh iceberg lettuce leaves.

Thai Chicken Soup with Rice Noodles

Ingredients:

- 4 cups chicken broth
- ½ cup shallots, thinly sliced
- 2 tbsp. Thai green curry paste
- 1 tbsp. vegetable oil
- 1 tbsp. fresh ginger, minced
- 2 tbsp. fish sauce
- 1 can coconut milk
- 4 heaped tsp brown sugar
- 2 tbsp. fresh lime juice
- ½ tsp turmeric
- 1 pack rice noodles

Instructions:

1. Heat the oil in a medium-sized saucepan or soup pot.

2. Add the ginger and shallots and cook for a few minutes, stirring constantly. Don't let the ginger burn.

3. Mix in the curry paste and cook for a minute.

4. Add the chicken broth, coconut milk, brown sugar, fish sauce, turmeric, and lime juice. Add salt if you wish to.

5. Bring to a simmer and gently cook for about five to six minutes.

6. While this is happening, make the rice noodles according to the instructions on the package.

How to Assemble

Adjust seasonings in the soup. Pour the soup over the rice noodles and gently give it a mix. You can serve this with cilantro or celery, and chopped scallions. You may also drizzle some Sriracha sauce over it.

Cauliflower Fried Rice

Ingredients:

- 2 lb. cauliflower
- 4 to 5 tbsp. vegetable oil
- 2 large eggs, beaten
- 2 scallions, chopped finely
- 3 garlic cloves, chopped
- 1 tbsp. freshly chopped ginger
- 4 tbsp. soy sauce
- 1 cup peas and carrots (frozen peas and carrots also work)
- ¼ tsp red pepper flakes
- 1 tsp honey
- 1 tsp rice vinegar
- 1 tsp sesame oil
- ¼ cup chopped cashews/ almonds/ peanuts
- Salt: As per taste

Instructions:

1. Grate the cauliflower, either by hand or in a food processor.

2. Heat the vegetable oil in a large skillet or cast iron pan.

3. Add the eggs and salt and keep cooking until the eggs are scrambled and cooked. Keep aside on a small plate. Carefully wipe the pan.

4. Again, add about 3 tbsp. of vegetable oil to the pan and keep it at medium heat. Add in the scallions, garlic, and ginger and cook gently.

5. Mix in the grated cauliflower, red pepper, soy sauce, honey, and salt. Keep stirring.

6. Then add the peas and carrots and keep cooking until the cauliflower is soft and the vegetables are tender.

7. After five minutes, add the rice vinegar, sesame oil, and nuts.

8. After about two minutes, add the eggs. Keep tasting and adjusting the seasoning.

9. Take off the fire and serve right away with a dash of soy sauce on top.

Thai Shrimp and Quinoa

Ingredients:

- 1 pound raw jumbo shrimp (cleaned, deveined and tail off)
- 2 cups chicken stock
- 1 and a 1/2 cups quinoa, uncooked
- 1 cup coconut milk
- 1 tbsp. coconut or any other oil
- 1 tbsp. fish sauce
- ½ cup small onion, chopped
- ½ tsp sesame oil
- 1 each, red and yellow bell peppers, chopped
- 2 medium carrots, julienned
- ½ tsp ground ginger
- Salt: As per taste
- 3 cloves minced garlic
- ¼ tsp red pepper flakes
- ½ a lime, chopped

Instructions:

1. Take a large cast-iron pan or skillet and heat the oil for a couple of minutes.

2. Add the fish sauce and sesame oil and stir.

3. After a couple of minutes, add the bell pepper, carrots, and onion and ginger. Add some salt at this stage.

4. Cook for four or five minutes until the vegetables become tender.

5. Now add the garlic and cook for another minute.

6. Add the coconut milk, quinoa, and chicken stock. Mix well, cover, and cook for almost 15 minutes until the quinoa is fully cooked.

7. Once done, remove the lid and add the shrimp to the mixture.

8. Adjust seasoning and add pepper flakes to it. Cover and cook for five to six minutes until the shrimp is translucent and cooked.

9. Serve hot with wedges of lime and a dash of cilantro on top.

Ratatouille Rice

Ingredients:

- 1 tbsp. olive oil
- 1 medium onion, diced
- 3 cloves minced garlic
- 1 medium zucchini, diced
- ½ eggplant, diced
- 1/8 tsp ground black pepper
- ½ tsp dried oregano
- ¼ tsp red pepper flakes
- 1 red bell pepper, diced
- 2 small tomatoes, diced
- 1 cup white rice
- 1 cup vegetable broth

Nicholas Bjorn

Instructions:

1. Take a skillet and warm the olive oil for a minute.

2. Add in the onion with a bit of salt, and cook until it becomes translucent and tender.

3. Add the garlic and cook until it gives off a nice aroma.

4. Now add the eggplant, zucchini, black pepper, oregano, pepper flakes, some salt, and stir. Cook this for about a minute or so.

5. Then mix in the tomatoes and bell pepper and cook until the tomato starts releasing oil and liquid around it.

6. Lastly, add the white rice and vegetable broth. Stir until combined and bring to a boil.

7. After a couple of minutes, simmer the mixture and cover and cook for about 18 minutes, until the rice is completely cooked. If you feel the rice is sticking to the bottom, add some more broth.

8. Check seasonings and add pepper, salt, herbs as desired. Serve this healthy dish hot from the stove, garnished with cilantro and basil.

Chapter 16 – Sweet Endings: Lip Smacking Healthy Desserts

So you thought desserts are the work of the Devil, full of rich and sinful things that you eat just once and repent at leisure? Do not fret. Here are some absolutely delicious desserts for you to indulge in, without going off the health wagon.

Avocado Chocolate Mousse with Summer Fruit

Ingredients:

- 4 ripe avocado

- ¼ cup coconut milk

- 4 tbsp. dark cocoa powder

- 3 tbsp. honey

- 2 ounces dark chocolate, melted (70 percent or more cocoa)

- 2 tsp vanilla extract

- 1/8 tsp salt

- Coconut whipped cream, strawberries, blueberries, and other summer fruit, chopped

Nicholas Bjorn

Instructions:

1. Peel and pit the avocado and put them inside a food processor.

2. Blend until well combined and creamy.

3. Mix in the cocoa, honey, milk, vanilla, chocolate, and salt. Keep blending until they mix properly. Taste at this point and add more honey if desired. The mixture should be completely creamy at the end of this.

4. Serving: Take out into pretty bowls and top with coconut cream or layer it with summer fruit such as berries, mangoes, even nuts and add a few nuts for extra crunch.

Raspberry Vegan Cheesecake

Ingredients:

For walnut crust

- 1 cup walnuts
- 3 dates (Mejdool or similar), pitted
- ½ tbsp. coconut oil
- ¼ tsp sea salt

For the raspberry layer

- 12 ounces frozen raspberries
- ½ tsp fresh lemon juice
- 2 tbsp. maple syrup
- 2 tbsp. chia seeds

Instructions:

1. Blend together the walnuts, salt, dates, and coconut oil in a food processor until the mixture turns crumbly.

2. Line an 8" by 4" loaf pan with parchment paper. You can also butter it beforehand. Press the crust onto the bottom and freeze until the next layer is ready.

3. Blend together the thawed raspberries, maple syrup, lemon juice, and chia seeds. The mixture should be smooth; no bits should be visible. Pour this mixture over the frozen walnut crust and smooth it out. Freeze this for at least four hours.

4. When you are ready to serve this dessert, take the cake out of the freezer and let it thaw for about twenty minutes.

5. Lift it out carefully from the pan. Slice into as many slices as you would like. Garnish with a sprig of mint for extra flavor.

Cinnamon Baked Pears

Ingredients:

- 2 pears, washed, cored and cut in half
- 1 tsp cinnamon
- 1 tsp maple syrup
- Pumpkin spice granola and coconut cream for toppings

Instructions:

1. Before doing anything, preheat the oven to 350 degrees.
2. Take a baking sheet and place the pears on it. It should stand straight on the paper. Or you may cut into any shape you desire or even bite-sized pieces.
3. Sprinkle it evenly with the maple syrup and cinnamon. Bake this for about 25 minutes.
4. Cool them and top with either the granola or any other nuts or berries and enjoy.

Healthy Peanut Butter Fudge

Ingredients:

- 2 cups finely shredded coconut
- 1 cup creamy peanut butter
- ½ cup coconut oil
- 4 tbsp maple syrup
- 1 pinch sea salt
- 1 tsp vanilla extract
- Toppings: peanuts, coconut flakes, nuts, etc.

Instructions:

1. First, line a 9" by 5" loaf tin with parchment paper.
2. Add the desiccated coconut to a food processor and blend on high speed until the mixture becomes creamy. Scrape down the sides and keep aside.
3. Add the peanut butter and coconut oil and blend one again at high speed.
4. Once done, mix in the maple syrup one tablespoon at a time. Check for sweetness and add until the desired level is reached. Don't add too much because then the coconut mixture with seize and you won't be able to work with it.

5. Add sea salt and vanilla extract and mix well.

6. Transfer this to the loaf pan or tin and spread it evenly all over. At this point, you can also add some crunch on top by putting nuts or flakes.

7. Now freeze this until it becomes firm. Take a knife and run it through hot water and cut the mixture into even squares. This will give you about twenty squares.

8. Serve immediately and enjoy it. You can also store these in the freezer for up to a month.

Nicholas Bjorn

No-Bake Brownie Energy Bites

Ingredients:

- ½ cup each walnuts and almonds
- 1 cup dates, chopped
- 1/3 cup plus 2 tbsp. unsweetened cocoa powder
- ½ cup shredded coconut flakes

Instructions:

1. Grind together the walnuts and almonds in a food processor. The mixture should form a dough.
2. Mix in the dates, coconut, cocoa, and a pinch of salt and incorporate it well into the dough.
3. Now, lightly grease your palms with coconut oil or use saran wrap to make balls out of the dough.
4. Roll these into the remaining coconut flakes or use corn flakes or almonds to coat the balls. Put them inside the fridge for a little while. Take them out and serve.

Apple Crumble

Ingredients:

- 5 apples, Granny Smith or similar
- ½ cup low-fat butter
- 3 and a half tbsp. flour
- ½ cup honey or maple syrup
- 1 lime
- 1 small stick cinnamon
- 1 tbsp. sugar
- Coconut cream: Optional

Instructions:

1. Preheat the oven to 180 degrees Celsius.
2. For the topping, take the butter in a plate and sift flour over it.
3. Add the honey. Mix these by hand until you get a crumbly mixture.
4. Peel the apples and cut them in half or bite-sized pieces. Place these in an ovenproof bowl.

5. Squeeze the lime over them and shake so that it is distributed equally, and the apples are not discolored. Sprinkle the one tablespoon sugar over them. Put in the stick of cinnamon over this.

6. When ready to go inside the oven, sprinkle the topping you just made over the apples. Bake for about 40 minutes, till the apple crumble turns golden brown.

7. Serve either hot or cold with coconut cream.

Yogurt Cocktail

Ingredients:

- 1 and a half cups yogurt or curd
- ½ cup plums
- 4 medium strawberries
- ¼ cup pineapple
- 4 tbsp. honey
- ½ tsp vanilla extract
- ½ cup non-dairy cream or coconut cream
- A few cornflakes- different flavorings

Instructions:

1. Chop the fruit into bite-sized pieces and put the mix in a big microwaveable bowl. Add some honey and microwave them on high for a minute.

2. Combine the yogurt, remaining honey, and vanilla in a bowl.

3. Add the coconut cream and mix well. Either put it in the fridge or strain through a muslin cloth to get rid of excess water and then put it in the fridge, depending on how you like the consistency.

4. Take the fruit bowl out of the microwave.

5. Layer the fruit one by one alternating with the yogurt mixture in a large glass bowl. For garnishing, use cornflakes or coconut flakes or any nuts of your choice.

Quick Coffee Dessert

Ingredients:

- 2 eggs
- ½ cup ground sugar or maple syrup
- A pinch of salt
- 1 tbsp. instant coffee
- 1 cup whipping cream or nondairy cream
- 2 tbsp. castor sugar
- 1 tsp vanilla extract
- ¼ tsp almond essence

Instructions:

1. Put the eggs, salt, and sugar in a bowl and beat with a hand mixer at high speed. The mixture will become lemony and fluffy.

2. Add the coffee and beat for a few more minutes. Keep this aside.

3. In another bowl, take the cream and sugar and whip until soft peaks form. It shouldn't be too runny or too stiff. Gently stir in the essences.

4. Fold the egg mixture into the cream and combine gently, making sure you don't lose the aeration.

5. Pour into individual glasses and freeze until you are ready to eat.

6. When serving, take the glasses out and let them sit for about ten minutes or so before digging in. If you wish, garnish with mint leaves.

Simple Rice Pudding

Ingredients:

- ½ cup rice washed and soaked in ½ cup low-fat milk
- 5 and a half cups low fat milk
- ½ cup sugar or honey
- Almonds: Blanched and slivered, a few
- Rosewater: A few drops
- Pistachios: A few

Instructions:

1. Blend the rice and milk, such that it becomes an absolutely smooth paste.
2. Take the other milk in a vessel and boil it. Pour the rice-milk paste and sugar or honey into it and continuously stir it on a low flame until the mixture thickens. Simmer for a while.
3. Take it off the fire.
4. Add the almonds and pistachios, along with the rose water and mix well. Pour into glasses or bowls and chill well. Serve with a glass of cold milk, if so desired.

Nicholas Bjorn

Rich Chocolate Slices

Ingredients:

- ½ cup butter or low-fat margarine
- 2 tbsp. honey
- 4 and a half tbsp. cocoa
- 225 grams semi-sweet biscuits
- 2 tbsp. raisins
- 2 tbsp. chopped mixed nuts

Instructions:

1. Mix the honey, cocoa, and butter in a pan and put it on a gentle heat. You will need to keep a watch over it and remove it as soon as the butter melts.

2. Mix the ingredients of the pan well and keep aside.

3. Meanwhile, crush the biscuits in a clean bag with a rolling pin or blend in a processor. You can do the same with the nuts. Keep aside.

4. When the butter mixture cools down, add the biscuit and nut mixture to it. Mix well. The final consistency should be crumbly, yet it should hold well when you compress it.

5. Grease a small cake tin with oil or butter and pour this mixture into it. Leave it inside the fridge to set.

6. For serving, let it rest on the countertop or dip the tin into hot water for a few seconds and invert it over a plate. Cut into slices and serve with fresh fruit on the side.

Nicholas Bjorn

Conclusion

If it wasn't clear from the beginning, stop chasing the latest diet trend and focus on the healthy weight loss and super foods in this book. Know that you can eat normally and still lose weight.

Your next step is to follow the strategies and recipes listed in this book. Apply what you have just learned. Take action and be consistent! The best thing you can do to lose weight and be healthier is to eat right.

Now, I would love to hear what you think! Please let me know if you enjoyed this book or what I could improve on. You can do that by leaving a review on Amazon. I'll be looking for your reviews when I come back to add more content my book. Thank you in advance!

Thank you, and good luck!

Nicholas Bjorn

Nicholas Bjorn

FREE E-BOOKS SENT WEEKLY

Join North Star Readers Book Club
And Get Exclusive Access To The Latest Kindle Books in
Health, Fitness, Weight Loss and Much More...

TO GET YOU STARTED HERE IS YOUR FREE E-BOOK:

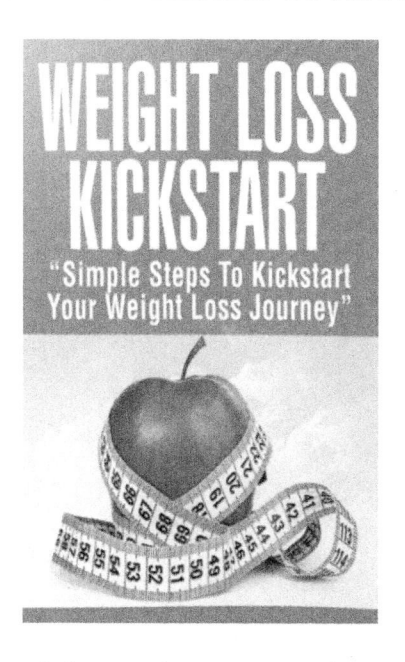

Visit to Sign Up Today!
www.northstarreaders.com/weight-loss-kick-start

Nicholas Bjorn

References

https://www.healthline.com/nutrition/top-10-evidence-based-health-benefits-of-coconut-oil#section10

https://www.ausnaturalcare.com.au/health/lifestyle/lifestyle/food/goji-berries-real-superfood

https://www.healthline.com/nutrition/11-proven-health-benefits-of-garlic

www.webmd.com

www.self.com

www.mayoclinic.com

www.nerdfitness.com

www.buzzfeed.com

www.tasty.co

www.healthline.com

www.jamieoliver.com

GOOD NUTRITION IS IMPORTANT – THIS IS A FACT.

BUT HOW DO YOU REALLY GET STARTED TO ACHIEVING IT? PEOPLE SAY IT BEGINS WITH A BALANCED DIET, BUT HOW EXACTLY DO YOU ACHIEVE THAT BALANCE?

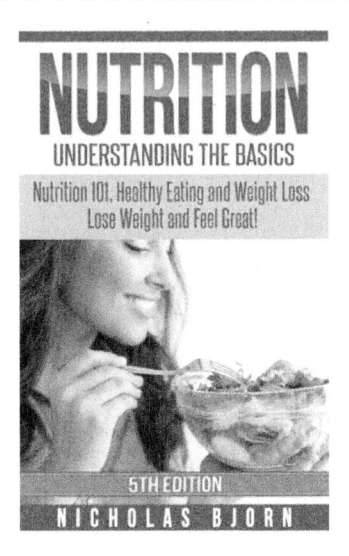

If you are lost in the world of calories and kilojoules, this book is the perfect reference to help you! The contents of this book will help you focus on what's important while getting rid of all the unnecessary fluff about dieting and healthy living that are just bound to confuse you.

Here is what this book has in store for you:
- Nutrition defined and simplified
- Dietary guidelines made easy to follow
- Nutrition labels made understandable
- Vitamins and minerals explained
- Fat-burning foods enumerated
- Meal planning and recipes made doable

Start reaping the benefits of eating healthy and living healthy! You can get started today.

Visit to Order Your Copy Today!
https://www.amazon.com/dp/1519485492

DO YOU WANT TO KNOW HOW YOU CAN LOSE WEIGHT AND BUILD MUSCLE FAST, STARTING RIGHT NOW? THIS BOOK WILL LET YOU IN ON THE SECRET!

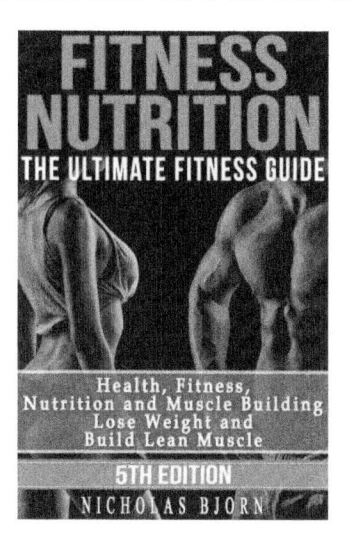

Everyone knows how important it is to maintain a healthy physique. Often, achieving the ideal body requires you to lose weight and build lean muscle. But how do you do that? To become physically fit, you need to have the knowledge necessary to get you on your way and the motivation required to keep you going.

Here's what this book has in store for you:
- Learn how your body uses calories and what role carbohydrates play in your weight
- Discover which foods contain good fats and lean protein that could benefit your body
- Determine what your meal frequency and caloric intake should be
- Know which exercises you should do to get that toned and sculpted look

With the knowledge you will gain from this book, you will be on your way to getting the amazing body that you want!

Visit to Order Your Copy Today!
https://www.amazon.com/dp/1514832968

Book 2

Weight Loss Motivation

The Ultimate Motivation Guide

Weight Loss, Health, Fitness, and Nutrition

Lose Weight and Feel Great!

3rd Editon

By Nicholas Bjorn

Nicholas Bjorn

© Copyright 2021 – All rights reserved.

In no way is it legal to reproduce, duplicate, or transmit any part of this document either in electronic means or in printed format. Recording of this publication is strictly prohibited, and any storage of this document is not allowed unless with written permission from the publisher. All rights reserved.

The information provided herein is stated to be truthful and consistent, in that any liability, in terms of inattention or otherwise, by any usage or abuse of any policies, processes, or directions contained within, is the solitary and utter responsibility of the recipient reader. Under no circumstances will any legal responsibility or blame be held against the publisher for any reparation, damages, or monetary loss due to the information herein, either directly or indirectly.

Respective authors own all copyrights not held by the publisher.

Legal Notice:

This book is copyright protected. This is only for personal use. You cannot amend, distribute, sell, use, quote, or paraphrase any part or the content within this book without the consent of the author or copyright owner. Legal action will be pursued if this is breached.

Disclaimer Notice:

Please note the information contained within this document is for educational and entertainment purposes only. Every attempt has been made to provide accurate, up-to-date, and reliable complete information. No warranties of any kind are expressed or implied. Readers acknowledge that the author is not engaging in the rendering of legal, financial, medical, or professional advice.

Table of Contents

Introduction 177

Chapter 1: How Motivation Works 181

    Phases of Motivation Needed to Get Things Done 181

    Motivation Suffers When You Hate the Activities 183

    Learning about the Fear that Paralyzes You 184

    External and Internal Motivation 184

    Surround Yourself with External Motivation 185

    Developing Pro-Health Principles 185

    Advantages of Focusing on Your Motivation 186

Chapter 2: Diet Challenges that Make You Hate Losing Weight 187

    Fear 187

    Paralyzing Self-Perception 188

    How Others Look at You 189

    Extreme Stress 189

    Overthinking about Weight Loss 191

    The Boredom Factor 191

    Presence of Food 194

Chapter 3: How to Boost Your Motivation to Maintain Your Diet Plan 197

    Maintaining Your Diet 197

    Your Weekly Meal Plan 198

    Preparing Your Meals 199

How to Make People around You Help in Your Weight Loss Goals 200

Weight Loss Motivation Techniques – Will These Work for You? 205

The Real Way to Get That Motivational Flow Going 208

Chapter 4: How to Boost Your Motivation to Work Out 211

How to Build Motivation for Working Out 211

Recharge Your Motivation to Exercise 214

Chapter 5: The Biggest Weight Loss Motivators 223

Diabetes/Pre-Diabetes 224

Improving Blood Sugar Control 225

Keeping Your Heart Healthy 226

Better Sleep 226

More Mobility and Less Pain in the Joints 227

Improvements in Energy Levels and Vitality 228

Improvements in Fertility 228

Chapter 6: Motivational Quotes 231

9 Things to Say to Yourself to Stay on Track 231

More Motivational Quotes to Help You Through the Day ... 235

Chapter 7: Tips to Help You Stick to the Diet 245

Avoid Skipping Breakfast 245

Eat Regularly 245

Eat More Fiber 246

Be Active 246

Hydrate 246

Read Labels 247

Use Smaller Plates 247
Stop Avoiding Foods 247
Avoid Stocking Junk Food 248
Reduce Alcohol Intake 248
Have a Meal Plan 248

Chapter 8: The Best Way to Start a Diet 249
Choose a Healthy Plan 249
Take Baby Steps 250
Set Realistic Goals 251
Use Rewards 251
Find a Buddy 252
Track Your Intake 252
Exercise! 252

Chapter 9: How to Stay Motivated 255
Define Why You Want to Follow the Diet 255
Set Realistic Expectations 256
Focus on Your Process 257
Choose a Plan that Suits Your Lifestyle 259
Maintain a Journal 260
Apps to Use as Food Journals 260
Find Support 266
Commit to the Plan 266
Ooze Positivity 267
Plan for Any Setbacks and Hurdles 268
Learn to Forgive Yourself 269
Appreciate and Love Your Body 270
Choose Activities You Enjoy 271

Choose Your Role Model 271

Get a Dog 272

Consult a Professional 272

Chapter 10: Morning Habits to Help You Lose Weight 275

Eat Protein-Rich Foods for Breakfast 275

Hydrate 276

Measure Yourself 277

Get Some Sunlight 278

Be Mindful 279

Exercise 279

Change Your Mode of Transport 280

Focus on Your Intake 281

Chapter 11: Small Lifestyle Changes to Lose Weight 283

Focus on the Portions 283

Pause Between Bites 284

Prepare Your Lunch 284

Focus While Eating 284

Snack Smartly 285

Sleep Well 285

Healthy Eating at All Times 285

Use Small Plates 286

Avoid Family-Style Eating 286

Do Not Face the Buffet 287

Eat Enough Vegetables 287

Chapter 12: How to Create a Customized Diet Plan to Help You Lose Weight 289

Step One: Do Not Use Calorie-Counting Diets 289
Step Two: Calculating Your Macros 291
Step Three: Find Foods That Suit You 292
Step Four: Find Every Recipe You Can 293
Step Five: Set a Schedule 294
Step Six: Track, Adjust, and Analyze 295

Chapter 13: How to Manage Your Weight Loss 297
Build Lean Muscle 297
Eat More Filling Foods 297
Curb Temptation 298
Count Your Calories 298
Meal Plans 298
Increase Your Activity Time 299
Watch Your Portion Sizes 299
Regular Weighing 299
Eat Dairy 300
Use Your Plate as Your Guide 300
Stop Watching too much TV 300

Chapter 14: Final Push – 21 More Ways to Remain Motivated 301

Conclusion 313

Resources 317

175

Nicholas Bjorn

Introduction

I want to thank you and congratulate you for purchasing this book, "Weight Loss Motivation: The Ultimate Motivation Guide: Weight Loss, Health, Fitness, and Nutrition – Lose Weight and Feel Great!"

This book contains proven steps and strategies to keep your motivation up while implementing your weight loss plan.

Anyone can lose weight if they put their minds to it. Unfortunately, there are factors around you that may sabotage your mind. These factors affect your motivation and, ultimately, your performance. The tasks involved in losing weight become easier if you know how to stay motivated. This book discusses how motivation will improve your performance. It also discusses how the different types of motivation play a part in your success.

The book also explains how the different states of mind may affect our motivation. Sometimes, it is our own state of mind that hurts our chances of success. This book helps you deal with these mindsets to increase your chances of reaching your weight loss goals.

It is difficult to lose weight, and it is even more difficult to change your lifestyle and diet plan so that you can meet your goals. You may be overwhelmed and may want to give up immediately. This happens to everybody, and this book is here to help you stop feeling that way. It will provide you with tips to help you create a plan for yourself that is easy to follow. It will also provide you with tips you can use to push yourself to do better and meet your outcome goals!

Once you begin a diet, it does become difficult to stick to it, especially if you do not have a plan in place. This book will leave you with some tips you can use to stick to your diet and find ways to motivate yourself to do better.

Lastly, the book gives tips and strategies for you to overcome common weight loss challenges. It provides pragmatic ways for you to surely reach your goals. These tips and strategies apply to both men and women.

I have also included lots of inspirational and motivational quotes, designed to give you that extra boost in motivation that you might sometimes need. The methods suggested in this book are proven to keep you enthusiastic and hopeful. You should start reading today to begin your weight loss journey.

Be warned that there are no quick fixes in this book. I am not going to give you a diet to follow, and I am not going to give you any exercise routines – that is for you to determine by yourself or with the help of nutrition and fitness experts. My goal is to give you the motivation you need to keep on going and succeed in your personal journey toward health, fitness, and happiness, as well as a slimmer you.

You need to understand and accept the fact that you are bound to make mistakes. You may want a cheat day in the middle of the week or binge on something you crave. This happens because of restricting your diet, and this is something you should not do. Focus on choosing the right means to lose weight, and reward yourself when you achieve your goals. Do not berate yourself for making a mistake, but start where you stopped.

Thanks again for purchasing this book. I really hope you enjoy it!

Weight Loss Motivation

FREE E-BOOKS SENT WEEKLY

Join North Star Readers Book Club
And Get Exclusive Access To The Latest Kindle Books in
Health, Fitness, Weight Loss and Much More...

TO GET YOU STARTED HERE IS YOUR FREE E-BOOK:

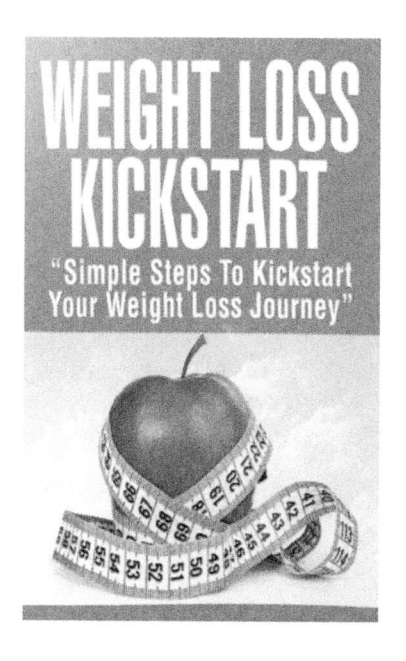

Visit to Sign Up Today!
www.northstarreaders.com/weight-loss-kick-start

Nicholas Bjorn

Chapter 1: How Motivation Works

Finding a source for your motivation is essential if you want to get things done. The most difficult things in life require a lot of motivation to accomplish. With an ever-increasing number of distractions and opportunities to procrastinate around you, it is difficult to keep yourself motivated these days.

The challenge of motivation is most evident in matters concerning health. Given that most health-related tasks that need to be done have no immediate observable effects, you may easily lose motivation to do them. In working out for instance, many people lose interest when they can't see any visible results after a few sessions. This causes some impatient people to look for shortcuts. Some of the weight loss shortcuts found in the market, however, have dangerous effects on your health. To avoid these types of workout methods and to keep yourself motivated, you must understand how motivation works.

Phases of Motivation Needed to Get Things Done

There are three major parts of workout tasks where motivation is essential; before starting, in the middle of the task, and before ending the task.

It usually takes a lot of motivation to start a health-related task. The amount of motivation you need is greater if you hate the activity. This is the type of motivation needed when you are trying to convince yourself to get out of bed in the morning to start running.

Many factors affect your ability to start tasks. You may not be confident in your skills to accomplish a task, and you may be planning to learn more before jumping in. It could also be because of underlying fears that cause you to procrastinate.

A lot of motivation is also needed when you are in the middle of the task. You need motivation to remain focused on your goal until you accomplish it. This challenge is most difficult when the task requires a lot of time before it is done. You will need a lot of patience to keep yourself focused on the task at hand and to prevent your skeptical mind from sabotaging your success.

The last phase of motivation is usually needed for the final push to get a task done. This phase of motivation prevents you from taking too many breaks when you are almost at the finish line. People are vulnerable to procrastination when they are already near the end of their goals because they think that only a small amount of work is needed to get the task done.

For most types of tasks related to losing weight, you will need these three phases of motivation to reach your goal. You need a lot of motivation to get off the couch and work out every day. You will also need motivation to limit your calorie intake and avoid high-calorie food types. When you are already in the middle of a workout and diet program, it takes a lot of motivation for you to keep pushing to get better.

Motivation Suffers When You Hate the Activities

After working out and dieting for a while, beginners tend to form a negative attitude toward these tasks. They tend to hate the pain and the sweat, and this leads them to procrastinate on their scheduled workouts and fail on their meal plans when they are confronted with delicious types of food. They tend to hate waking up for a morning run or getting ready to go to the gym.

People cite a lot of reasons why they hate tasks related to losing weight, but you'll be surprised by how far off these are from the primary reason. The most basic source of all our hatred toward these tasks is fear. Your mind can become a victim of modern types of fear. These fears are the biggest factors that demotivate you even before you start.

In losing weight, one of the most common challenges is the fear of failing. If you have tried losing weight in the past and you failed at some point, you already have thoughts of failure ingrained in your mind. When you try to do the same task in the future, this lingering fear will remain in your mind. It will come out and do damage on your motivation when you are most vulnerable.

For most people, this is when they are in their beds, and they feel that they deserve to be resting. This is the time when you usually ask yourself: "What's the point?" You begin to question your whole motive for working out.

Given the strong effects of fear on you during this weak mental state, you need to learn how to control your own motivation. You need to be constantly aware of your level of motivation. As long as you do this, you will have the strength to carry on in your weight loss journey.

Learning about the Fear that Paralyzes You

Motivation is not just about pushing through against laziness. It is also about dealing with the fears you already have in your mind. Every time you are about to skip on a scheduled workout session or every time you place too much food on your plate, you should ask yourself these questions: Why am I doing this? What am I afraid of?

In the process of answering these questions, you will be able to reflect on your present attitude, and this will lead to keep working on your goal. By analyzing your thought process, you will not only prolong your motivation but also build a state of mind that allows you to control it.

As Zig Ziglar said, motivation is not permanent. Even if you succeed in boosting your motivation today, you will need to do it again tomorrow. That is the nature of motivation. You have to constantly work on it. You can do this by using both internal and external sources of motivation.

External and Internal Motivation

This process of self-reflection will help you develop strategies to help increase your external and internal motivation. External motivation is the type of motivation derived from sources outside of your mind. This is the type of motivation you experience when you feel like working out because you hear one of your favorite workout songs. The people and things that surround you affect your external motivation. Although this type of motivation is easy to create, it doesn't last very long. You should use it together with internal motivation.

Internal motivation happens when the principles and values you abide to become the reasons behind your actions. If you have this type of motivation, you do not need to hear any type of music just to start working out. Although this type of motivation is more difficult to develop, you should still work on it because its effects last longer. To have a strong source of internal motivation, you need a combination of two things: constant motivation practice and a set of positive principles to follow.

Surround Yourself with External Motivation

In the beginning of your weight loss program, it is understandable that your internal source of motivation may not yet be strong. In the early stages, you will need to make sure that the people and things around you motivate you to work harder. You should also decrease the factors that demotivate you in your surroundings. Tell your family and friends what you are doing so that they can encourage you to continue. Post a journal of your daily food and exercise regime on your Facebook page so that your friends can keep on pushing you to carry on. Only buy healthy foods; instead of heading for the cake section in the grocery store, head for the fruit section.

Developing Pro-Health Principles

Good health is a principle everybody should abide by. Unfortunately, many people take this aspect of their life for granted. It becomes a secondary priority next to finances and careers. If you want to lose your excess weight and keep that weight off, you need to develop a pro-health principle. This means that you want to lose weight because it is good for you. You are not working out and dieting just to look good, but you are doing so because of all the benefits that it brings to your life.

You will be able to develop this principle by constantly reminding yourself of the positive things that a healthy life can bring. For instance, by losing your excess weight, you will live longer, and you will have more time to enjoy with your family. If you love your job, losing weight and becoming healthier will allow you to increase your working hours on your projects. Keep focusing on your weight loss, and you will eventually develop this life principle.

Advantages of Focusing on Your Motivation

By learning how to focus and improve your motivation, you will learn a lot about yourself and how your mind works. You will not only learn about your fears but also where they come from and their particular effects on your behavior.

Motivation is a game changer. If you have tried and failed at losing weight in the past, learning about your motivation and practicing the principles offered in this book will significantly improve your chances of success.

By being aware of how motivation works, you will also develop a no-excuse mindset. Knowing that you can control your motivation prevents you from placing too much emphasis on uncontrollable factors in reaching your goals. You will hold yourself accountable in all your failures, and you would only have yourself to thank for all the successes that you gain.

Chapter 2: Diet Challenges that Make You Hate Losing Weight

Losing weight is not easy. There is a lot of muscle pain and sacrifice involved. If you haven't had any personal victories when it comes to losing weight, there are a lot of challenges that will make you lose motivation. You should be aware of these to prevent them from having too many paralyzing effects on your mind.

Fear

One of the biggest challenges is fear. You can try to avoid your fears, but doing so only strengthens them. The right way to deal with your fears is to identify and face them. Most modern fears are all in the mind. Many of them are not actually warning us from danger, as they should. Most of them only succeed in making us avoid new experiences. This is the nature of modern fears.

However, not all fears are bad. Some of them are rational. These types of fear warn you that your life may be in danger if you carry on with what you are doing. There are some types of fear, however, that have nothing to do with survival at all.

After identifying your fears, you need to separate the ones that are rational from those that are unnecessarily paralyzing you.

For most types of fear, the best way to deal with them is to constantly put yourself in experiences where you can face them. These experiences will desensitize you from the factors that you fear. As your mind becomes accustomed to working with these factors, it will no longer generate the sensation of fear every time you are about to face the same experience.

Paralyzing Self-Perception

Some types of fear also lead to a distorted way of seeing yourself. People who think of themselves as incapable of reaching their fitness goals sabotage themselves from reaching success. They surrender even before starting the battle.

For people who have this kind of self-perception, the first step is always to accept it. The usual reaction when someone points this out to them is denial. They tend to deny that their self-perception is the main factor that prevents them from even signing up to the gym or creating a diet plan. Accepting your self-perception is the first step to changing it.

After accepting this fact, the next step is to build your self-esteem by winning personal victories. Personal victories are the foundations of a healthy self esteem. You could start by taking on small weight loss-related tasks. When you achieve success with these tasks, you should write them down in a list. As the list of your personal victories become longer, you will become more confident to take on more difficult tasks.

How Others Look at You

For some people, their fear of being judged by others affects their actions too much. They fail to follow the plan in times when their mind becomes occupied by how other people think of them. People with this type of fear are prone to overeating when they are with a group of people who make fun of their attempt to lose weight.

The people around us can be mean. They ridicule people who are trying to lose weight because of their own failure to do so. They make other people feel horrible because deep inside, that's how they feel about their own weight and health problems. As you may have noticed, most fit people like talking about how they remain fit. This is not because they are self-centered but because many of them like to motivate others to do the same. A fit person feels bad every time they see someone they love suffering from weight issues.

You can deal with your fears, but you will not be able to change the negative attitude of others. However, you can control the people that you surround yourself with. If someone makes you feel bad for trying to lose weight or influences you to eat more than you should, avoid them at your time of weakness. In times when you are feeling down and your motivation is low, you should surround yourself with people who will lift your spirit and help boost your motivation.

Extreme Stress

If your mind is preoccupied with seemingly important thoughts and these thoughts cause you to become stressed out, you may not have the focus to continue on your workout and diet plan.

There are two approaches when dealing with these types of stress. You could deal with the cause of your stress first before continuing to work out, or you could try to stick to your plan even in the face of great mental stress.

In the beginning of your weight loss journey, you will have a hard time continuing on your weight loss plan when you are facing a great deal of stress. If this is true for you, you should do the first suggestion above. There are some types of people, however, who feel better when they work out. The good feeling that follows after working out helps in coping with the source of stress. If you are this type of person, you should do the second suggestion stated above.

You could schedule a session or two with a massage therapist to help relieve stress, or you could take up yoga and make it a part of your routine. Yoga not only helps you to get incredibly fit, but it can also help you clear your mind of the stresses and strains of each day.

Meditation is another great stress buster. It can teach you deep breathing techniques that you can do at any time and in any place. These techniques will help to eliminate any stress that you may be feeling. It can teach you to redirect your focus onto positive energies and banish the negative energy from your life. Meditation can be done for as little as five or ten minutes at a time, enough to help you feel refreshed like a new person and with your motivation levels fully intact.

Overthinking about Weight Loss

The mental toll of reaching your weight loss goal can also become a source of stress. When the stress caused by overthinking about weight loss becomes too high, it may also cause your motivation to work out to dwindle.

Success in weight loss can be achieved if you are doing the tasks needed to be done without spending too much time thinking about them. This is where mindfulness becomes useful. Mindfulness is a state of mind where you are only focused on one thing. The thing that you focus on should be the task at hand.

When it's time to work out for instance, you are only focused on that task and nothing else. It is inevitable for thoughts about your work or finances to creep into your mind. For very important thoughts, you need to have a piece of paper and write them down in a list. The less important thoughts, on the other hand, should be released. The idea is to get your focus back on the task at hand as soon as possible.

The Boredom Factor

The boredom factor is the single largest reason why people fall off their diets and lose the motivation to continue. It is all too easy to look at your diet sheet and see nothing more than a list of restrictive foods. Let's face it; there is only so much plain chicken or boiled fish you can eat, and who wants to eat green leafy vegetables all day long? Who wouldn't get bored with a diet sheet like that?

The answer to boredom and the best way to give your motivation levels a boost is to get creative with your food. Go to the store, and stock up on spices, herbs, fresh fruit and vegetables and then start looking for good ways to bring them into your meals. The following are just a few ways that you get creative with your food and really look forward to meal times:

- **Spice Things Up**

Spices and herbs are an excellent way to pep up your food. Instead of plain old chicken, add some fennel and rosemary. Rub mint into your next pork chop, and coat fish in lemon, mint, and pepper. If your food is bland, the spices and herbs will have a fantastic effect, giving them a completely different taste. So, don't be afraid to experiment.

- **Dress it Up**

A nice fruity vinaigrette is a great marinade for your meat or a lovely dressing for your vegetables – hot or cold ones. Try sprinkling a bit of raspberry vinaigrette over your broccoli or apple cider vinegar and pepper over your cabbage.

- **Infuse Your Olive Oil**

Instead of plain old olive oil, try infusing it with some of your favorite herbs and spices. Try adding a clove or two of garlic, a couple of sprigs of rosemary, or a few basil leaves to a bottle of oil. Red or green chili peppers or red pepper flakes do just as well, too. Leave the oil for a while to allow the flavor to infuse, and you'll find that it gives your food a real boost in flavor. Use it for sautéing or in your favorite healthy salad dressing to give it a bit of zing.

- **Soy Sauce**

This is especially true for the low-sodium kind. This makes a fantastic addition to any food. Sprinkle a few drops on your meat or over your vegetables. Add it to a healthy stir-fry or in with your rice as it's cooking. Soy sauce adds a little bit of extra flavor to anything, and there is little that it will not work with.

- **Make it Fruity**

Those dark green leafy vegetables that taste so bitter at times can taste wonderful with fruit. Serve up your spinach with raspberries, chunks of fresh pineapple, or segments of mandarin orange, and I guarantee you'll never shy away from a dark leafy vegetable again. Blend spinach or kale with fresh fruit to make a healthy and tasty smoothie, or dress it up with a fruity vinaigrette.

- **Make it Different**

Instead of serving up chunks of zucchini, spiral it instead, and use it as a healthy alternative to pasta. You can spiral carrots, cucumbers, any type of squash, or parsnips – you name it. You could sauté zucchini and carrots that have been spiraled and add a few olives, capers, and Italian tomatoes for a tasty Italian meal without the calories.

When you start to get bored with your food, instead of falling off the wagon and heading back to the cookies, simply change things up. Experimentation is the key here; see what works and what does not. Not only will you enjoy doing it, but you will also start to look forward to meal times again.

Aside from the mental aspects that prevent you from reaching your goals, you should also consider the external factors that may affect your motivation negatively. Here are some of them:

Presence of Food

You can't just rely on your willpower to avoid the temptations of food. Everybody has a breaking point when it comes to temptations. Your willpower should only be the last line of defense. You should actively decrease the amount of time that you are exposed to food while you are still developing the discipline to resist it. This means that you should choose the types of events that you go to socially. Avoid social events that encourage you to pig out.

There are some types of events, however, that are just too important to avoid. If you need to attend events like these and there are a lot of tempting foods in the venue, you should make sure to stay in areas that lessen your interaction with these foods. You should engage with people, for instance, to occupy your mind. Before you know it, the event is over, and you haven't taken a single bite.

There are also some food types that you just want to try because of taste. These are the types of food you want to try even if you are not hungry. In this case, you should not be afraid to take a small piece, and take just a few bites. The real challenge is not taking a second serving. You could use the "avoidance" strategy suggested above after you have taken your first bite.

Nicholas Bjorn

Chapter 3: How to Boost Your Motivation to Maintain Your Diet Plan

We already touched on some parts of this topic in the last section of the previous chapter. In this chapter, we will discuss more strategies and scenarios where your motivation to avoid eating and lose weight will be put to the test.

Maintaining Your Diet

People usually eat more than their fair share when they haven't planned their food source for the day. Office workers are prone to this problem. They are usually absorbed in their jobs, and they don't give a lot of thought to the sources of their food. This makes them reliant on unhealthy food sources, such as preserved food products or fast food.

You can avoid these food sources by planning out your meals throughout the day. You will have a stronger chance of resisting food temptations if you are not hungry most of the time. To do this, you should evenly space your meals throughout the day.

The ideal meal plan is to eat 6 small meals in your waking hours. Most adults eat 3 big meals and countless snacks in between. After eating one of their big meals, they will probably feel hungry again after 2 hours. As it is not yet time for another big meal, they snack on the available food sources around them. For most people, the basis for their food choices is the taste. Tasty foods are usually high in fats and calories. You can avoid choosing these by creating a weekly meal plan.

Your Weekly Meal Plan

Before the week begins, you should plan the types of food that you will eat throughout the week. By doing this, you will be able to plan what to buy from the grocery store and adjust the number of calories you consume according to your fitness goals. A person living a sedentary lifestyle will need 1800 to 2600 calories per day. Women and older people generally need lower amounts.

To know how many calories to consume for you to lose weight, you should write down a list of foods that you eat daily for one week and calculate the corresponding number of calories that you consume each day. You could have a nutritionist do this for you if you are not sure how many calories each food type has. Alternatively, for detailed information on how calories work and how many daily calories you need, you can check out my book "Fitness Nutrition" https://www.amazon.com/dp/1514832968

It is easy to decrease the number of calories that you consume if you take away the unhealthy types of food from your diet. You should be aware of the food types that are high in calories. If you eat these types of food, you will eat too many calories before becoming full. Some of these food types are chocolate, cheese, sugar-filled drinks, nuts, and dried fruit. A handful of chocolates, for example, is equivalent to 2 cups of rice in calories.

Preparing Your Meals

Keep in mind that we are trying to avoid instances where you need to rely on preserved and fast foods in your meals and snacks. To do this, you will need to prepare your own food each day. It is highly suggested to prepare your food for the whole day every morning. You should follow the daily prescribed number of calories when preparing your meals. The next step is to divide the food that you prepare into six servings, and place them into vacuum-sealed containers to preserve their freshness.

The average person is awake for 16 hours a day. That means that you should eat your meals every 2 and a half to 3 hours. If you want to avoid eating before you sleep, you could modify the process by eating only 5 times a day. You will eat slightly bigger meals, but the number of calories that you consume will still be the same.

By following this plan, you will reduce the number of calories that you consume at one time. Your body will have more time to digest the foods that you consume, and by the time you eat your next meal, your body will have already digested the majority of the previous meal.

As your meals are evenly spaced, you will not become hungry in between meals. This will lessen your unhealthy snacking and prevent you from relying on fast foods and high-calorie packaged foods. You will be satisfied most the time, which means that you will have stronger willpower to resist offers of food.

How to Make People around You Help in Your Weight Loss Goals

Let People Know about Your Goal

You should tell the people around you about your plan to lose weight. Most people will understand and adjust their behavior towards you. If they know that you want to lose weight, they are less likely to offer you foods you are avoiding and support you in your food choices. This will also help them understand why you have a different meal schedule.

Document and Track Your Progress

If you let the people around you see your progress, it will help them understand your point of view. Creating a blog or posting your personal weight loss victories on your social media accounts is a great way to motivate you and keep you focused on your goals. Your friends who understand your goals will be supportive, further boosting your motivation.

Avoid People Who Sabotage Your Success

There are some types of people who will make fun of your effort. You should try to avoid insensitive people who will only make you feel bad. They usually undermine your effort and make you lose your motivation. They could also be the types of people who fill your head with negative thoughts. These are the people who constantly keep saying that you can't do it or that what you are doing is not important.

Hang Out with Supportive People

Surround yourself with people who share the same goals and concerns. You should find people who are also trying to lose weight. These are the types of people who congratulate you for your small victories and give you consoling words in the face of failure. They know how you feel because they are facing the same challenges. They will also be happy to have you around because your motivation also boosts theirs.

The following are tried and tested motivational strategies to help keep you on the weight loss track.

1. Look for more than a single source of motivation

If there is one way to keep you motivated on your weight loss journey, it's to find more than just one single reason to stay motivated. Some of the motivations that you could use to make sure you stick to a healthy diet are:

- You feel full of energy
- You jump out of bed in the mornings instead of pulling the duvet over your head
- You are at your ideal weight, and you want to stay there
- Your stomach is no longer bloated
- You enjoy food without suffering painful indigestion
- Your skin looks brighter and clearer

It's up to you to figure out what would motivate you to keep on eating those wholesome healthy foods and stay away from the bad stuff. Sit and think about it, make a list, and use that list as your means of motivating yourself.

2. Set long-term goals

Most people think only in the short term when it comes to losing weight, and many of their goals are unrealistic. The quickest way to lose motivation is to set a goal where you want to lose, say 10 lbs. in two weeks. First off, that is not a healthy way to lose weight and keep it off, and second, it is not really attainable, and when you see after week 1 that you've only lost 2 lbs., you'll realize that and your motivation is gone.

Long-term goals really are the difference between failing and succeeding. Weight loss itself is a short- or medium-term goal, but you need to look beyond that. Think about what you want to do when you get to your target weight. Maybe there is a particular activity you've always wanted to do but couldn't, maybe you want be able to run around after your children or your grandchildren, and maybe your goal is that you want to stay healthy and free of disease until your long healthy life comes to an end.

3. Take it slow

When you make the decision that you are going to lose weight and suddenly switch from doing little exercise and eating a poor diet to eating healthy and going into training, it can be something of a shock to your system. You will need to learn how to prepare food in a different way, how to eat more vegetables and fruits, and maybe even how to shop properly, and your body is going to react hard to a sudden change. It needs to learn how to digest these new foods and how to stop craving addictive foods for a start. The harder your body reacts, the more likely you are to give it all up, so the best thing to do is ease yourself in. Give your mind and body a chance to adjust to your new way of life, and you will be more likely to hang on to the motivation to succeed. Keep this in mind – it doesn't matter how fast you make changes; what matters is that you do, and you stick with them for the long term.

4. Find treats and comfort foods that are healthy

When you first make the change to a healthy diet, you might feel a little lost. The simple reason is that you are used to eating your favorite treats – those comfort foods are what you turned to in times of need, so you are feeling a bit empty, as if there's a big void that needs to be filled. There are plenty of healthy treats and comfort foods that can fill that void. If you have a sweet tooth and tend to turn to chocolate, simply puree up a banana and some cocoa powder with some ground flax to make a healthy chocolate pudding.

5. Keep things simple

You don't need to prepare complicated gourmet meals every day. Yes, it is nice to take time preparing a meal and making it look good, but for most meals, you can stick to basic foods like steamed vegetables and rice, a baked sweet potato, or a soup. Just use those herbs, spices, and vinaigrettes I talked about earlier to spice things up in simple ways. Find meals that you really enjoy, and just make a few simple changes to keep them interesting.

6. **Never feel guilty**

It takes time to make the transition from an unhealthy diet to a healthy one, and it is important that you do not get obsessive over what you are doing. Stress causes an awful lot of problems health-wise, and it is important that you do not stress yourself out over what you eat. Nobody can stick to a healthy diet every single day; we all have days where we give in to temptation. The important thing is that you don't feel guilty over it, and you don't use it as an excuse to slip back into old habits. Guilt is a negative emotion, and it simply makes you eat more to feel better about yourself. Don't punish yourself by eating less or exercising harder and longer because that won't work either. Simply take each day as it comes, and move on. If you slip up, simply pick yourself back up, and carry on with your new healthy diet.

7. **Stay positive**

Positive energy is the key to realizing your goals. Unfortunately, most people tend to focus so much energy on avoiding the bad stuff that they miss out on the fun of trying new foods and the effects that a good nourishing diet has on your body. Find healthy foods that you love to eat like fruits, some nuts, or a special healthy dinner. Eat them as often as you can so that you maintain a positive attitude, and keep that positive energy flowing through you.

Weight Loss Motivation Techniques – Will These Work for You?

Think tortoise and hare when you think of diets and losing weight – it really is slow and steady that wins. So, to keep you motivated and inspired to carry on, have a look at these common techniques for motivation, and ask yourself if they would work for you.

- **Sticking motivational quotes to your mirror**

Visual reminders are never a bad thing, so ask yourself if putting some motivational quotes on sticky notes on your mirror would help you. You can actually stick these notes anywhere – the fridge or in your car – just as little daily reminders about what you are trying to achieve.

- **Weight loss jars**

Visualization techniques are some of the best ways to keep yourself motivated. Get two jars – clear ones because you need to see what's inside them – and some colored pebbles or glass balls. Put one pebble or ball into one of the jars for every pound that you weigh, and for every pound you lose, take it out of that jar and put it in the other one. A quick glance is enough to tell you how well you are doing.

- **Food Labeling**

It's one thing to pack up your lunch and your snacks for the day, but what if you are tempted to eat it all in one sitting? Putting labels on the containers with the time you are meant to eat the food and how many calories are in the food can help you with portion control.

- **Leave your workout gear out and ready for use**

It can be difficult to walk past a mat that's been left unrolled without getting down to do a couple of crunches or a few yoga poses, but you could go one step further. Leave a set of hand dumbbells in your bedroom, perhaps a resistance band or an exercise ball in the lounge, and your running shoes by the front door as way of reminding you that exercise is important.

- **Buy some of your clothes in the next size down**

While it's always good to think about how you are going to lose the weight, it's also good to think about how you are going to look when you have lost it. So, prepare yourself for your weigh-in, and buy a few clothes that are the next size down. Hang them where you can see them when you wake up and when you go to sleep.

- **Pin a "fat" photo to your fridge**

Find the worst photograph of yourself, and pin it to your fridge door. This way, whenever you feel tempted and head to the fridge, it's the first thing you see. This should be motivation enough for you to leave the candy in the fridge and pick up an apple instead.

- **Share your food journal**

Everyone tells you that, when you are trying to lose weight, you should keep a journal of everything you eat. That's all well and good, but it doesn't stop you from failing. What you might do is opt to share your food journal with someone else. You can either email it to a close friend or family member who you know is going to support you, or you can go all out and publish it on your social media pages for all your friends to see.

- **Dress in your workout gear first thing every day**

Even if you are not intending to head out for a workout straight away, wearing the clothes is a great way of making sure that you will get out of that door and go for a run instead of finding an excuse not to.

- **Lolly sticks**

Write down all your fitness and diet goals on lolly sticks – for example, 25 crunches, walk 2 miles, etc. – and put them all in a plastic cup. Pull one out and complete it, and then put the lolly stick in another cup. Label the cups appropriately so you can see how much you have done and how much is left to do. As one cup begins to empty and the other starts to fill, you will find yourself even more motivated to keep going.

- **Always have food with you**

Diets do not have to be restrictive. In fact, those that are restrictive are the ones that you are more likely to give up on. Being on a diet isn't necessarily about cutting down on the amount you eat; it's about changing what you eat, and going hungry is not a good motivator. Always have food with you – a couple of bits of fruit, a tub of chopped up carrots, peppers and celery, or a low-fat yoghurt. This way, when you get the munchies, you will not be tempted to head for the bakery and pick up a double chocolate chip muffin with a side order of chocolate chip cookies. You will have food to eat – healthy snacks that will keep you full and satisfied – and keep the cravings at bay. Knowing that you are not about to go hungry and fall into temptation is motivation enough to keep going.

The Real Way to Get That Motivational Flow Going

- Don't choose to focus on positive or negative fantasies about your future self. Instead, focus on both. Doublethink everything, looking for the bad side as well as the good.

- Do train yourself to realize that, at some point, your willpower is going to disappear. Instead of wallowing in misery, tell people what your goals are, and ask for support to lower the chance of you failing

- Don't stick to picking a goal; pick all of the sub-goals as well. The goal is what you want to achieve, and the sub-goals are how you are going to achieve it.

- Look for the right role model. If you are scared of failing, then look for a role model who has failed. It is their story that will inspire you to succeed.

- Don't ever beat yourself up if you eat something that's not allowed. The power of regret is far more powerful if you use it before you do something or if you fail to do something than it is if you wait until afterwards.

- The most important thing is to realize that no motivational technique on earth is a magic pill. They can't make you lose weight – only you can do that and, if you don't really want to succeed, then you won't. If you do want to succeed, then you have taken the first step, and these motivational techniques will help you.

Nicholas Bjorn

Chapter 4: How to Boost Your Motivation to Work Out

There are two major components of weight loss: your diet and your daily activities. To lose weight, you should eat just enough food to keep you energized for your daily activities. We discussed that in the previous chapter.

In this chapter, we will focus on building your motivation to keep exercising. Maintaining an active lifestyle will increase your metabolic rate. It will make your body burn more energy even while you are resting.

To be able to integrate workouts into your lifestyle, however, you should make sure that you enjoy them. If it feels too much like work, it will be too difficult to maintain. There will come a time that your mind will be defeated by the distractions and temptations around you.

How to Build Motivation for Working Out

Set Realistic Goals and Make a Plan to Reach Them

Before you can start lifting weights, jogging, or doing other types of activities, you should put in writing what you want to achieve. If you want to lose weight, you should set the exact number of pounds that you want to lose and the amount of time that you have to achieve your goal. You could also set your goals for specific body parts like your waistline or your arms.

Following the SMART philosophy for setting goals is an ideal tool to use. This ensures goals are specific, measurable, attainable, realistic, and have a timeline. You should then find a workout plan that fits your schedule and your personality. You should consider the time that you have for your workouts and the effort that you can devote to it.

Remind Yourself of the Benefits of Working Out

Being aware of the benefits of working out will help you continue doing it. You will also be able to build your willpower to avoid being lazy. This will remind you that you are not doing this just to look great but also to become healthier.

Make a List of Activities that You Enjoy

If you love dancing, you should include that into your workout plan. If you prefer sports, you should train for the type of sport that you want to participate in. By doing things that you like, you will be able to transition to an active lifestyle with much more ease.

Include a Variety of Activities in Your Workout Plan

Aside from doing what you love, you should also make it habit to try new things and to vary the activities in your workout plan. Lifting weights or running all the time will become boring after some time. If your body is not presented with a challenge every so often, it will no longer improve.

Prepare the Necessary Equipment and Outfits

Spending for your workout plan is like investing in your body; you will be expecting a return on your investment. Not only will you feel like an athlete, but this will also make you work harder and become more disciplined in following your strategies.

Make Your Workouts a Social Activity

You should avoid doing everything by yourself. Just like in your diet plan, you should also include the people around you. Join people who also like working out. Motivation, enthusiasm, and positive thinking are contagious. You will have a better chance of continuing your weight loss program if you have these people around.

Analyze the Factors that Motivate You

You should also use your metacognitive abilities to improve your performance. Every time you feel extra motivated, you should analyze the internal and external sources of your motivation.

Being aware of these factors will give you insight into how your mind works. You can use some of these factors to stimulate your motivation when you are feeling down.

Reward Yourself for Reaching Your Goals

Rewards are things that you allow yourself to have when you achieve a certain goal. They are expected to increase the likelihood that you will repeat your positive behaviors. You should decide on the rewards that you will give yourself when achieving your goals. The thought of the reward will help motivate you. In times when the workout routine becomes difficult, you should remind yourself of the reward that you will get if you push through.

You should make sure, however, that you will be able to follow through with your promise. The most important promises are the ones that you give to yourself.

Recharge Your Motivation to Exercise

The only thing that is standing between you and the body you want is mental block, so to get over those speed bumps and avoid the inevitable excuses, follow these top methods for rebooting your workout and your mental and emotional state.

Weight Loss Motivation

You Think – My scales are stuck, why am I bothering?

Rethink – This pudge will go.

Stick with it. Weight loss is never consistent, and the scales, unless they are cheap or faulty, will never lie. First off, the more weight you have to lose, the quicker it will come off – IN THE BEGINNING. After that, it will all start to slow down. Most people reach a weight loss plateau, where they don't lose any weight for several weeks, and it is at this point that you must not give in.

One more important point – do not weigh yourself every day; it's a very bad habit. Your weight will go up and down daily, but it will go down overall. Weigh yourself once a week or fortnight. That way, any loss in weight is a much bigger motivator. Weighing yourself daily is the best way to demotivate yourself, so don't do it. Just because you aren't losing any pounds doesn't mean that your body isn't losing inches, and the only way to tell that is how your clothes fit. Give yourself plenty of credit for how much better you look, and use that as your motivation to continue.

Redo – Move your routine up a notch.

As you lose weight, your metabolism will adjust to accommodate the lighter, smaller you. That means you are going to have to change the way you encourage your body to burn fat and shed pounds. If you are already on a light diet of around 1500 calories a day, don't cut any more off. Instead, make your workouts more intense, and work out for a bit longer each time. Not only will this result in more calories being burned off, but it will also make your cardio capacity much larger. This means that you will find it easier to exercise and will be motivated to work out for just a little bit longer. Crank up the resistance on the stationary bike, set the treadmill at more of an incline, walk for a bit longer than you do now, walk at a faster pace, or go for one-minute interval runs. Between toning exercises, fit in a set of jumping jacks, running on the spot, or step-ups.

You Think – I really can't manage another rep.

Rethink – Don't my biceps look fantastic!

If you need a motivational boost or a bit of a lift, psych yourself up mentally and emotionally while you are training. This can increase your muscle power by up to 8%, as well as their size. Bigger muscles result in an increase in metabolism, which burns off fat faster. So, if you needed just one bit of motivation, there it is.

Mental imagery is a wonderful boost – when your arms or legs feel tired, imagine bigger and stronger muscles and tell yourself how great you look; you will get another rep or two out.

Redo – Take it down a notch.

If you really can't manage another rep at the same rate, lighten things off a bit. If you are lifting weights, knock the weights down by 10% until you know you can do another rep in good form. If you are sprinting circuits, slow it down for the last one. The more effort you put in, the better the rewards will be, so even if your final rep is at a lower rate than the previous ones, it's still more effort, and it will reap rewards. Don't ever beat yourself up if you can't do it, but keep this in mind: Pushing your limits a little further will get you results you never dreamed of seeing.

You Think – I can't run a mile!

Rethink – That jogger looks like Brad Pitt/Angelina Jolie – whoever takes your fancy at the time really!

When you are slogging your way through that mile, turn your thinking to what is going on around you. Yes, you may slow down a little, but you will keep on going, and you will finish that mile. Repeat a mental mantra over and over again – something like, "I am a running machine" – and you will find that you can go for longer and further.

Redo – Divide and conquer.

If you are running a mile, to start with, split it up into some running and some walking. Jog for maybe quarter of a mile, and the walk for a further half mile before jogging the final stretch. As you get better and fitter, as well as leaner, you can jog further and gradually cut down the walking time. If you can do this three times a week, it won't take long before you can run the entire mile. Your motivation? Your fitness and how you look. Think about how much better you feel, and you will keep on going. Do set up a routine for running, though. If you only go when you feel like it, it will not work.

You Think – I've damaged my knee/leg/arm, etc., so I won't be able to do any exercise for a month.

Rethink – Where did I put that Pilates DVD?

If you injure yourself and stop working out, it takes a maximum of three days for your body to start losing its conditioning. If that isn't enough motivation of you to get up and go, tell yourself this: There's more than one way to reach that goal. Start by making a list of all the negative thoughts you are having, and then turn them into positive thoughts. For example, "I can't go to my exercise class tonight; everything I've done will all go to waste," could be turned into, "Oh well, now I can start using that Pilates DVD I bought."

Redo – Switch things out.

Your regular exercise class might be out, but there are other options that are low or no impact. Depending on what injury you have sustained, a bit of moderate training on the elliptical bike can burn off up to 416 calories an hour, and water jogging can burn 512 calories an hour, as can cycling. These are all good alternatives but only if your injury allows it. If you can't exercise because your legs are injured or you have knee pain, you can still exercise the upper part of your body with hand weights. You can still sit on a chair and punch a boxing bag. Also, Pilates is a form of exercise that is gentle yet effective – designed to allow the maximum benefits in a safe way.

You Think – Spinning classes are way too intense for my liking.

Rethink – That guy over there in the Lycra shorts doesn't look as tough as he thinks.

We are afraid of the unknown – of what we don't know – so before you dismiss a particular exercise, have a go at it. You might just find that you enjoy it. Watch a class first, right from the start. If you see a spinning class from the middle onwards, the pace and the sweat are going to put you off, but if you see it from the beginning, you might just find that it is not that bad.

Redo – Find your own pace.

With most exercise classes, you are in control of how it makes you feel. Just because the rest of the class is throwing themselves about or the other runners on the track are sprinting all the way does not mean that you have to. If there comes a point in the class where the instructor tells you to increase resistance, only go as far as you are comfortable going. If you get tired and can't keep up, slow things down a bit. The idea of exercise is to get the hang of it while doing it correctly and safely and to have fun. Go into each class telling yourself that you are there to enjoy yourself, and you will.

You Think – I can only exercise at home; that's not going to work!

Rethink – There really is no place like home!

The first thing you have do is work out what is going to motivate you to get off the couch and stay off it. Then, you need to come up with a plan that is going to put you in the frame of mind to commit to exercising at home. Put your workout clothes on when you get home from work or first thing in the morning so that you get in the right mindset and know you are going to exercise. Create a schedule that has accountability in it. For example, get a friend to come around on certain days, and do those kickboxing or fitness DVDs.

Redo – Get a takeaway.

I don't mean the fast food one. If you can't afford to join a gym, you can have one beamed into you lounge for a fraction of the cost. Using email and website, personal trainers are there to help you without you having to leave your own home. Some of them will provide you with a customized routine to follow, as well as a diet plan.

You Think – I can't stay on that cardio machine for more than 30 minutes; it's like a form of slow torture!

Rethink – Who's going to be sent home tonight on BB/Jungle/X-Factor, etc.?

When you are on the treadmill, don't waste your time thinking about the exercise you are doing; it won't work. Instead, turn to other things, like watching your favorite TV program or plugging into your music and losing yourself in it. You might just be surprised at how fast the time goes and how much more you achieve when your mind is elsewhere.

Redo – Work first, rest later.

Plan your routine so that you start hard and fast and slow down towards the end. If you start off with high-intensity workouts and then go on down to lower intensity, especially on the treadmill, you will find that more fat is burned, and your workout won't feel quite so stressful. Your motivation is that you know you can finish light and not be absolutely worn out, dripping sweat, and feeling like you couldn't move another step if you wanted to. Try this 45-minute plan – warm up for 5 minutes at a nice, easy pace. Increase speed up to a moderate level, and for 20 minutes, increase your speed or incline by 1% every 2 minutes. Then, lower the incline and/or the speed slightly for 15 minutes, followed by 5 minutes at a nice, easy cool-down pace.

You Think – I haven't got the energy to exercise after work.

Rethink – Just 10 minutes, that's all!

There is a huge difference between mental and physical tiredness. Believe it or not, physical activity can knock down your mental fatigue. Tell yourself that you will do just 10 minutes, and you will find, more often than not, that you end up doing more, simply because once you get going, your tiredness and fatigue disappears. Not only that, but your mood improves, too.

Redo – Stack it in your favor.

When you leave work to go home, make sure your route goes past your gym. The sight of people exercising is often motivation enough, so make sure you have your workout gear with you. Not only that, but you can also give yourself a big pat on the back for having taken time out to exercise instead of going home and flopping down on the sofa.

If you don't feel like doing a full gym workout, have an alternative plan in place. Get off the train or the bus a stop earlier, or have your workout mat already set up in front of the TV and the workout DVD ready to go. If you have an alternative plan in place, you are twice as likely to have the motivation to work out, and you are twice as likely to actually do something instead of opting for the easy way out.

It is very easy for me to tell you to learn to see things in a more positive light, but that is exactly what you have to do. When something negative pops into your mind, change it into a positive thought. Think of another way of doing something. If you really can't get to the gym, exercise at home instead of giving it a miss altogether. Tell yourself that you can do those extra few minutes and that you can push yourself that little bit further.

Nicholas Bjorn

Chapter 5: The Biggest Weight Loss Motivators

The single biggest motivator anyone should ever need for losing weight, eating a better diet, and working out more is their health. Obesity is a contributing factor to many different health conditions, and losing just 5% to 10% of your weight can result in massive benefits, both short and long term.

If sufficient weight can be lost to bring your body mass index back into a safe range and so that you are no longer classified as clinically obese, the benefits will be even bigger.

Some of the heath conditions caused by being overweight are:

- Type 2 diabetes
- Pre-diabetes
- Heart disease
- Arthritis, osteoarthritis, and other joint pain-related conditions
- Infertility

Losing weight can help you to:

- Avoid diabetes and control your blood glucose levels better
- Keep your heart healthy
- Sleep better
- Move better and eliminate pain in the joints
- Have better energy levels and feel more vitalized
- Have much better fertility

Let's look at each of these in turn:

Diabetes/Pre-Diabetes

Pre-diabetes is caused by high blood glucose levels, and this occurs when the glucose levels are much higher than normal, but not high enough that you can be officially classed as having diabetes. Type 2 diabetes is when the pancreas no longer produce sufficient amounts of insulin to meet the needs of your body, or the insulin that is produced is not doing its job properly. If you have pre-diabetes, you have a much higher chance of getting full-blown type 2 diabetes later on.

One of the leading risk factors for diabetes is obesity. Having to carry the excess weight makes it very hard work for your cells to respond in the proper way to the insulin that your body produces. This is because the fat that you carry is acting as a layer of insulation, and this makes it hard work for sugar to get into the cells. This results in more sugar or glucose circulating through your blood than there should be.

If you are diagnosed with pre-diabetes, you can work on preventing it from turning into type 2 diabetes by losing weight and keeping it off. Recent studies showed that if obese people were to lose 7% of their weight and do moderate activity, such as walking for a total of 150 minutes per week, they can either delay or prevent the onset of diabetes by around 58%.

Improving Blood Sugar Control

Excessive levels of sugar in the blood that is not controlled properly mainly cause complications in diabetes. The risk of suffering from chronic heart disease, heart attack, stroke, blindness, kidney failure, and even amputation of the legs is much higher for a person with type 2 diabetes, and this is as a direct result of the excessive sugar levels attacking the blood vessels and damaging them.

By controlling the levels of glucose in the blood, diabetic patients can prevent, or at least delay, some of these complications from occurring, but just lowering the level isn't enough. It has to be maintained and controlled very tightly, and one of the best ways to do this is to lose weight and get involved in a healthy eating and regular exercise program.

Keeping Your Heart Healthy

High blood pressure and high cholesterol are the two biggest risk factors for heart disease. Recent studies have found that when excess fat accumulates in the body, it will release chemicals that occur naturally into the bloodstream. These chemicals cause a rise in blood pressure, and the excess weight is what causes the liver to produce too much LDL cholesterol.

LDL cholesterol, or low-density lipoprotein, is known as bad cholesterol. It is sticky, and it settles in the blood vessel walls, which leads to the arteries narrowing down, causing a condition known as atherosclerosis. It is also a leading risk factor for stroke and heart attack. When a person loses weight, blood pressure tends to go lower, and the levels of LDL produced by the liver are reduced. The results from a study at the Royal Adelaide Hospital showed that a 10% reduction in LDL levels, a 12% reduction in total cholesterol levels, an 8% reduction in systolic blood pressure, and a 5% reduction in diastolic blood pressure could be achieved with weight loss.

Better Sleep

Overweight people are more likely to snore than those who are not overweight. Snoring is caused by the airways narrowing down, which obstructs the movement of air. Overweight people have a lot more soft neck tissue, which can increase the chances of snoring. However, snoring may also be one of the symptoms of a condition that can be life-threatening. I am talking about sleep apnea, a condition in which the person's airway is obstructed completely, causing inability to breathe. To start breathing again, the person has to wake up.

A person who has sleep apnea can wake any number of times throughout the night but will rarely remember doing so. The sleep and the oxygen deprivation can cause devastating health effects, including a severely compromised immune system, high blood pressure, heart disease, memory problems, and sexual dysfunction.

Losing weight can cut down on the amount of soft tissue in the neck and reduce snoring, and maintaining a good weight can encourage you to sleep better and reduce the risk of sleep apnea.

Studies have been conducted to see the effect of weight loss on how severe sleep apnea is, and it was found that losing 10% of your weight can decrease the level of sleep apnea events by 26% every hour. A further study was conducted obese people with type 2 diabetes and sleep apnea. It was found that those who reduced their weight were more than three times more likely to almost completely eliminate their sleep apnea episodes compared to those who did not lose any weight. Those who lost more than 10 kg in weight showed the greatest reduction of episodes per hour.

More Mobility and Less Pain in the Joints

Osteoarthritis is one of the most common joint disorders. The condition causes the bone and the cartilage that protects the joints to wear down; as a result, the joints can become tender and swollen. This can make movement painful, and being overweight will exacerbate this by putting more stress on the joints, especially the hips and knees. When you walk, an estimated force of between three and six times your weight is placed on the knee, so carrying an extra 10 kg in weight can equate to between 30 and 60 extra kilograms.

Losing just 5% of your body weight can cut down the stress on the hips, knees, and lower back and significantly cut down on pain. Remember that losing just 5 kg will equate to a reduction of between 15 and 30 kg of stress on these joints. In a loss of 10% of body weight, it has been shown that the symptoms of knee osteoarthritis can improve by 28%.

Improvements in Energy Levels and Vitality

When a person loses weight, we know that the physical levels are easily seen, but what many people do not think about is the psychological benefits. Studies have shown that when weight is lost, a person will benefit from a better quality of life, higher levels of energy, higher self-esteem, and lower rates of depression. This, in itself, is one of the greatest motivators.

Improvements in Fertility

It has been shown though numerous studies that obesity can have a serious effect on fertility and reproduction. Although the exact nature of the relationship between the two has not been shown, it is thought the excess of body fat can cause ripples in metabolizing the sex hormones that are responsible for the menstrual cycle.

It has also been reported that obesity during pregnancy can increase the chances of miscarriage and medical complications. Specifically, pregnancy-induced hypertension, gestational diabetes, thromboembolism, preeclampsia, and sleep apnea are the conditions most likely to occur.

In addition, deliveries for women who are obese may be further complicated by increased rates of caesarian section, labor induction, and a difficult labor because of the size of the baby. The babies born to overweight or obese women have a much higher rate of being admitted to neonatal intensive care and having congenital defects. Injuries during birth and fetal death are also more likely in obese cases, and babies are likely to have a much heavier birth weight, which puts both the baby and the mother at risk of trauma. The baby may also go on to suffer childhood obesity and possibly lifelong obesity.

Although there have been few studies conducted on the reproductive implications of losing weight in obese women who have problems with fertility, one study did show that even a small loss in weight for an obese woman who is infertile can raise the rate of ovulation, rate of pregnancy, and successful outcome of pregnancy.

Nicholas Bjorn

Chapter 6: Motivational Quotes

Motivation really is the key to success in anything, and diet, fitness, and weight loss are not exceptions to that rule. This chapter is all about getting motivation in a different way – through inspirational quotes and through telling yourself that you will succeed.

9 Things to Say to Yourself to Stay on Track

Everyone makes mistakes, especially when it comes to sticking to a healthy lifestyle, but whether you missed a few workouts (or a lot) or you completely fell off your diet wagon, it doesn't take very much to get yourself back in the saddle again. All you need is motivation, and one way to get that is to surround yourself with inspirational quotes.

Whenever you read them, they should help you to channel that energy and to stay positive, banishing negative thoughts from your mind altogether. These are just some of the quotes you could write down on sticky notes and pop around your home or office for a little motivation when you feel you need some.

"Being defeated is only a temporary condition. Giving up is what makes it permanent."

You now that you were only going to pick up a cup of coffee to take to work this morning, but that muffin really did call out to you. When you fall prey to a craving, it could just be the temptation you need to ditch your diet for the rest of the day. Don't. Having one muffin is one thing, but throwing your healthy eating plan away and eating whatever takes your fancy for the rest of the day is not the answer. Savor that muffin, and then get straight back on track.

"Strive for progress, not perfection."

How many times did you hit the snooze button this morning? That last time meant missing out on your morning workout, but while you could probably give yourself a good kick, bear in mind that your entire weight loss and fitness goal does NOT depend on that one workout. Tomorrow is another day and another chance to work towards your goal. If you really feel that bad about it, fit in a walk at lunchtime or after work. In a few months' time, when you look back on your journey, you won't even remember the time you couldn't to the gym.

"Fall down 7 times, get up 8. Don't give up!"

For most of you, this definitely will not be your first time on the diet roundabout. Some people simply can't succeed on their first attempt, and it might take several. If you really do struggle to stick to a clean-food diet or just can't find the time to get to the gym, don't worry about it. The next time you try could just be the time when it all falls into place.

Weight Loss Motivation

"Yes, you can! The road may be bumpy, but stay committed to the process."

You've been dead good; you've been to the gym and followed your routine on time every day for weeks, and then you bust your back. So, you can't get to the gym or do your normal routine for a few days, but hey, that doesn't mean sitting back and doing nothing. Go for a gentle walk, and then cook up a good healthy meal. Healthy lifestyles are made from lots of things, not just one, so don't give up when you come up against a stumbling block.

"Optimist: Someone who figured out that taking a step backward after taking a step forward isn't a disaster; it's more like a cha-cha."

Every day, the numbers on your scale go up, and then they go down, but you know, that's fine. This is all about living a healthier life, being happier and fitter, and not just about getting into that pair of skinny jeans you wore 5 years ago. Setbacks are everywhere in life, and you just have to deal with them, whether its missing out on a workout or giving in to temptation at the vending machine because you didn't have time for lunch. While you should always have your short-term goals in mind, you should always have your focus firmly on the long-term goals.

"It's how you handle the mistakes that creates your success."

So, all day long, you've stuck with the plan and eaten all that lovely healthy food. Then, you go home and fell into a block of cheese while you were making dinner. Don't beat yourself up over it. Instead, see it as the motivation you need to make improvements. You know when you will be at your most vulnerable to giving in to temptation, so make sure you are prepared for it. Have a healthy snack on hand to eat on the way home so that you don't walk through the door starving.

"Stay committed to your decisions, but stay flexible in your approach."

You are the one who made the commitment to leading a healthier life, but that doesn't mean that you are in control all the way. You can eat clean foods when it's you doing the cooking, but what about when you go out for a meal or to relatives who only eat packaged and processed foods? Instead of getting annoyed that you can't stick to your healthy diet, go with the flow and make the commitment to get back on track the next day.

"If you stumble, make it part of the dance."

So, you've given in and opted to try a new diet craze, but after a couple of days, you've already stumbled. This diet isn't for you because there is no way on earth you are giving up the cream in your coffee. Instead of throwing in the towel straight away, look at the diet as a whole. Is there any way that you can make that concession if the rest of the diet is going to work for you? Work out what you want and what your mind needs, and then stick to it.

More Motivational Quotes to Help You Through the Day

One of the most famous motivational quotes is: "Motivation is what gets you started, but habit is what gets you going." This is an accurate representation of how motivation fits into diet and fitness. Without it, you will not get the results you want, even if you follow a diet to a tee and stick to your fitness routine. The following are ten of the very best motivational quotes in the world.

"You can do it, even if it takes some time!"

"A huge part of losing weight is believing you can do it and realizing that it isn't going to happen overnight."

Weight loss and self-confidence are interlinked. When your confidence is high, you find it easier to lose weight because you believe in yourself. When you lose that weight, your self-confidence grows will grow because you will feel better. Believing is the force that drives you, but patience must be your guide. You don't lose weight overnight; it takes time. After all, you didn't gain it all overnight, did you?

Nicholas Bjorn

"No More Excuses."

"No more excuses.

No more negative body thoughts.

No more, 'I'll do it tomorrow.'

No more sitting and wishing for a thinner me.

No more eating when I am not hungry.

No more waiting for this to get easier.

No more muffin tops.

No more wobbly thighs.

No more soft, round stomach.

No more 'buts...'

No more 'I can't...'

No more 'it's too hard...'

No more 'I'm too tired...'

NO MORE EXCUSES."

You know that there is no end to excuses that you could come up with as to why you can't start your diet just yet or why you can't make it to the gym. Excuses are for losers, and it's the winners who make and take the opportunities. When you find yourself thinking up an excuse, turn it around, and make it into something that you know you will be proud of tomorrow.

"What you do is who you want to be."

"The difference between who you are and who you want to be is what you do, and what you have to do to get where you want to be may not be pretty or may not come easy."

We fall into two categories – people who want more out of life and those who are happy to settle for a little less. When it comes to losing weight and getting fit, aim high, or you will get far less. Make your goals higher to gain greater benefits.

"No pain, no gain."

"No, your legs aren't that tired. Yes, you can breathe. Keep going."

The famous Muhammed Ali was once quoted as saying, "No, I don't count my sit-ups; I only start counting when it stars hurting because they're the only ones that count." Always aim to do more and push your limits. Get through the pain barrier, and the benefits will flow.

"Challenge is a step forward."

"If it doesn't challenge you, it doesn't change you."

If you ever find yourself in a situation that is a little unusual, it is because you are challenging yourself and your abilities. To go from spending your life slouched on a couch to being a top fitness fanatic is the biggest challenge you will ever face, so step up and take it on.

"Love yourself, and respect your body."

"I don't work out because I hate my body; I work out because I love it."

If you want to change the way your body looks, you must first accept it as it is now. Love your body, love how unique it is, and use your workouts to improve on it.

"Make the first step today."

"Every journey begins with a single step, but you'll never finish it if you don't start."

Pythagoras once said, "The beginning is half of the whole." When you take that first step, what follows will become easier. You have to take that first step though because you cannot finish something that you haven't started.

"Work for it."

"Don't wish for it; work for it."

While that first step is important, in order for you to be able to take it, you have to work hard for it – it isn't going to happen with a wave of a magic wand. In health and fitness, you have to work for your results and work hard; otherwise, your wish will stay exactly where it is now and will never become a reality.

"Are you a weight loss winner, or weight loss loser?"

"Winners find a way; losers find an excuse."

Which category do you want to be in? Are you with the winners or the losers? Think about it carefully, because it is as simple as that. You decide what you want to be and set the targets, or you claim defeat and walk away.

"Where do you want to go tomorrow?"

"You can feel sore tomorrow, or you can feel sorry tomorrow. You choose." – Unknown

Whatever you achieve today will be what sets up your feelings for the next day. Make your choice. Do you prefer to feel disappointed or satisfied? You need to make the decision today, because tomorrow, you may not be in the right frame of mind.

"Do What's Best for You."

"If you don't do what's best for your body, you're the one who comes up on the short end." – Julius Irving

What this comes down to is this: If you don't look after yourself, you will end up coming up short. Everything will suffer – your health, your body, and your mind, and ultimately, that means you will. You don't have to.

Nicholas Bjorn

"Can't isn't the answer."

"Instead of giving myself reasons why I can't, I give myself reasons why I can." – Unknown

Put simply, "can't" is not a word that should be in your vocabulary, so eliminate it today.

"Don't give up."

"Never, never, never, never give up." – Winston Churchill

One of the most motivational speakers, Churchill came up with one of the simplest sentiments ever. Simply, don't ever give up, and don't ever stop trying.

"Always visualize."

"You must begin to think of yourself as becoming the person you want to be." – David Viscott

This is one of the truest motivational quotes ever. You should always see yourself as how you want to be, who you want to be, and how healthy you want to be.

"Try, and try again."

"The difference between 'try' and 'triumph' is just a little umph!"
– Marvin Phillips

This quote highlights how important it is to work hard and be determined because the end is worth the work.

"To your health!"

"The groundwork of all happiness is health." – Leigh Hunt

Healthy people are happy people. In working towards your weight loss goal, make health improvements your very first milestone because this will be what sees you through to end.

"Act now!"

"The time for action is now. It's never too late to do something."
– Carl Sandburg

How easy it is to put something off until tomorrow, but sometimes, tomorrow never comes. If you are struggling to get started, use this quote as a mantra you could keep repeating to yourself. Sometimes, we only get now to make a choice, so do it while the opportunity is there.

"Don't quit!"

> "The man who can drive himself further once the effort gets painful is the man who will win." – Roger Bannister

At the end of the day, the only person you are competing against is you, but you should still keep this quote in mind. Losing weight is tough, and some days are harder than others, but when you give it all you've got – when you use all that will power and all that self-control – the rewards are great.

"Don't feel inferior."

> "No one can make you feel inferior without your permission." – Eleanor Roosevelt

While Eleanor Roosevelt had a lot of wise things to say, this is perhaps one of the wisest. We all know that obesity carries its own stigma, but it really doesn't have to. You do not have to let anyone make you feel bad about anything

"Mind over matter."

> "The good Lord gave you a body that can stand most anything. It's your mind you have to convince." – Vince Lombardi

This is perhaps one of the truest quotes ever because losing weight really is a case of mind over matter. If you feel thinner in your mind, you can think your way to being thin. Getting it straight in your mind is the beginning of your journey – from there, it gets easier.

I hope that at least some of these quotes will give you the motivation you need to continue on your journey. It is hard, but it is a rewarding journey. Regardless of the blips you may encounter along the way, keep these quotes in mind to give you the motivation to continue.

Nicholas Bjorn

Chapter 7: Tips to Help You Stick to the Diet

It is difficult for anybody to change their lifestyle, and it is especially hard to stop eating the food you love to eat or even control what you eat. This chapter will look at some tips you can use to help you stick to your diet.

Avoid Skipping Breakfast

You do not lose weight if you skip breakfast. If you skip breakfast, you may miss some essential nutrients in the morning, forcing you to snack throughout the day because you are hungry. Having said that, if you choose to follow the intermittent fasting eating pattern, you can skip breakfast. Bear in mind that you need to stick to the eating pattern if you want to lose weight easily.

Eat Regularly

It is important to eat meals at regular intervals to burn calories faster. When you eat regular meals, you can reduce the temptation you feel. You can curb your cravings and manage your hunger pangs.

Eat More Fiber

It is important to increase your fiber intake if you want to improve your metabolism and reduce your hunger pangs. Fruits and vegetables are the best foods to include in your diet because they are low in fat and calories. They are also rich in fiber. These three ingredients are important if you want to lose weight. Fruits and vegetables both contain a lot of minerals and vitamins.

Foods with fiber keep hunger at bay. This is a good idea, especially if you want to lose weight. Fiber is found in most foods that come from plants, such as oats, brown rice, beans, lentils, peas, fruit, and vegetables.

Be Active

You need to stay active if you want to lose weight. It is especially important to do this if you want to manage weight loss. Exercise not only helps you lose weight but also has numerous benefits. It can help you burn any excess calories you eat throughout the day as well. If it is difficult for you to exercise regularly, choose an activity you love.

Hydrate

People are often thirsty when they feel pangs of hunger. You often consume too many calories when you could have stopped the hunger pangs by drinking a little water. So, ensure you drink enough water throughout the day to ensure you are not thirsty.

Read Labels

It is important to read food labels to ensure you choose the right options for you. Suppose you want to determine if you can consume a certain type of food; learn how to use the calorie information on the food label. Use the information to determine the effect of some foods on your weight loss.

Use Smaller Plates

If you want to reduce the quantity of food you eat, stick to using smaller plates. When you use smaller bowls and plates, your body will adapt and get used to eating smaller portions. You can sustain yourself throughout the day without feeling hungry. Your stomach takes 20 minutes to tell your brain that it is full. So, chew slowly, and do not eat any more food if you feel full.

Stop Avoiding Foods

If you ban foods from your diet, you will crave those foods. Do not remove foods you like from your diet. Banning only increases your craving because this is how your mind works. You can enjoy treats occasionally, but be sure to stick to your caloric intake.

Avoid Stocking Junk Food

You can avoid temptation if you do not stock junk food. You cannot eat too many biscuits, chocolate, and crisps. It is best to avoid soda and other carbonated drinks. Choose healthy snacks instead, such as unsalted rice cakes, fruit, oat cookies, popcorn, or juice. You can drink fruit or vegetable juice, but do not add too much salt and pepper.

Reduce Alcohol Intake

You may want to drink a glass of wine when you eat dinner. Did you know that one glass of wine and a piece of chocolate have the same number of calories? If you keep drinking a glass of wine during each meal, you are bound to gain weight.

Have a Meal Plan

It is best to plan your meals, including your snacks, for the entire week. Ensure you stick to your caloric intake and requirements. It is best to create a weekly shopping list and buy everything you need over the weekend.

Chapter 8: The Best Way to Start a Diet

It is a good idea to start a diet to lose weight because this improves your health. It is a worthy objective, but it is overwhelming to change everything about your life. You will face challenges when you begin anything new, and it is harder if you need to do this multiple times a day. This chapter has some secrets and tips to help you lose weight and keep that weight off. After all, what is the point of losing weight if you are only going to gain it all back again?

Choose a Healthy Plan

It is important to identify the right plan, and stick to it. This plan should include foods you love, along with other foods, such as vegetables, fruit, low-fat dairy, whole grains, seafood, lean meat, nuts, and beans. These foods have fewer calories when compared to other foods that can satisfy your cravings. These foods can help you stick to your diet and are rich in fiber. They are also low in fat and have enough protein.

You will slowly stop craving your favorite food, especially those high in calories and fats. A diet will help you control your intake of heavily processed foods and replace those foods with nutritious and healthy options. Bear in mind that you can change the foods you eat and the plan you follow if you need to. You can switch some foods for others if you want. You can change your plan at the end of a week or month, depending on how you feel.

Do not worry if you have intolerances, allergies, or are a vegetarian. You can include all the food groups recommended for you in your diet, but ensure that whatever you add provides the required nutrition. It is recommended that you take a multivitamin or mineral supplement in case you have any nutritional gaps.

Take Baby Steps

It is hard to change, and it is best to make small and gradual changes. Experts recommend that you change only one thing every week, so your body and mind get used to the idea of things changing. The objective is for you to develop and establish new habits that you can sustain for a lifetime.

The easiest way to do this is to stock your pantry and refrigerator with foods you should consume on your diet. You also need to plan your meals and eat something healthy. If you are unsure of what foods you can cook, buy a cooking magazine or cookbook specializing in a specific cuisine. If you still are not satisfied, join an online forum where people are discussing similar issues. Something on those websites is bound to help you.

Set Realistic Goals

It is hard for people to lose weight because they set unreasonable targets. They dream about fitting into old clothes or into clothing sizes that are not realistic. If you lose even 5% of your body weight or more, it changes the way you feel. You will find yourself motivated to do better and improve your health and wellbeing. Losing even a little weight helps to lower your blood sugar, cholesterol levels, and blood pressure.

It is best to set goals that are realistic and attainable. Experts recommend that you lose only one or two pounds each week. If you lose more, it is a sign of unhealthy weight loss. Bear in mind that slow and steady is the only way to go. It will take time for you to learn new eating habits, especially if you want to follow these for the rest of your life.

Use Rewards

As you maintain realistic and attainable goals, it is easy to meet them in the required time. It is best to reward yourself every time you reach a goal. If you exercise five times a week or lose five pounds, you need to pat yourself on the back. Find simple and effective ways to reward yourself.

You also should never be too hard on yourself if you cannot stick to your diet plan. It is important to remember that everybody has trouble with sticking to a new eating plan. If you do fall off the wagon, find a way to get back on track. Use this situation to identify what foods cause you to stop following your diet, and decide how you will take care of yourself in such situations without giving up. Experts recommend that you break the rules

20% of the time and adhere to them 80% of the time so you feel healthy.

Find a Buddy

It would help if you had someone to support you when you begin your weight loss plan. You can ask a friend or family member to support you. They may not want to partake in the diet plan, but you can ask them to work out with you or take a walk. If you do not want to ask your friends or family for help, join an online forum, and connect with people on the same journey. These people will be your source of support, encouragement, and inspiration. You can speak with them as often as you can, and it is better to have this support, especially when things get tough for you.

Track Your Intake

You need to know how much you eat in every meal. You need to document this to keep your intake in check. Write it down so you can control yourself. Use a diary or an application or tool to track your intake. Most applications give you a chance to measure your intake and track your consumption of nutrients.

Exercise!

I cannot emphasize this any more. Bear in mind that cutting your caloric intake and eating healthy is only a part of your success. If you really want to lose weight, you need to be active.

Weight Loss Motivation

Through exercise, you not only lose weight by burning calories but also increase your coordination, strength, and balance. This reduces stress and improves your health and wellbeing.

It is best to get some exercise every morning, but ensure you do not overwork yourself. Do not squeeze in a workout in between your hectic schedule because this does not work for most people. Before you begin any new activity, speak with your doctor. You also need to discuss your eating plan to ensure you provide your body with enough nutrition to sustain you throughout the day.

Be proud of yourself. It is hard to change your lifestyle and eating patterns, and you should pat yourself on the back for making this decision. Bear in mind that the road ahead will have a lot of potholes and bumps, but if you have a good plan, the right attitude, and a support system, you are going to succeed.

Nicholas Bjorn

Chapter 9: How to Stay Motivated

Have you started a diet recently but could not stick to it for longer than a week or maybe a month? Well, you are not the first person to go through this. The idea of sticking to a new diet plan or lifestyle does seem impossible, but this only happens if you do not have the motivation.

If you look back, you can determine exactly when you stopped following the diet. Now, if you think about the situation, you know you were no longer motivated to follow the diet, so you gave up. You can find different ways to motivate yourself, and this chapter includes some of the best ways to do so.

Define Why You Want to Follow the Diet

It is important to define why you want to lose weight. Grab a notebook, and make a note of these points. Keep this sheet close to you so you stay committed. This list will also motivate you and help you reach your goal. Read through this list regularly, and use it as a reminder, especially when you feel like straying from your plan.

You may have many reasons, such as keeping up with your kids or grandchildren, preventing the onset of diabetes, improving your self-confidence, looking great at an event, or fitting into your best clothing. Most people begin their weight loss plan when their doctor suggests that they lose weight. Research shows that people often lose weight faster if they are motivated for reasons that do not relate to a doctor.

Therefore, define your objectives or goals, and make note of them. Ensure you drive yourself to meet your goals because of how you feel from within.

Set Realistic Expectations

Most diet products and diets claim you can lose weight easily. Some may even help you lose weight in a week or two, but this is not healthy weight loss. Experts and nutritionists recommend you lose anywhere between 1 and 2 pounds a week. If you lose more than that, it is an indication of unhealthy weight loss. It is best to set attainable goals to avoid frustration. If you tell yourself you need to fit into a specific dress in less than two weeks, you are going to be annoyed.

When you set achievable goals and accomplish them, you feel a sense of accomplishment. Meeting self-determined and set goals often push you to work harder, and you are bound to lose more weight and stick to the diet plan for the long term.

A study conducted by Grave R D et al. in 2005 was based on weight loss data collected from different centers. According to the research team's analysis, women who did not set realistic goals and objectives often dropped out of their weight loss programs. The good news is that even a small loss in weight can go a long way. You will feel better after losing even a little weight. For instance, if you are 180 pounds and lose 18 pounds in 9 weeks, you will feel a lot better than you did a few weeks ago.

When you lose even 5% of your body weight, you can:

- Reduce the risk of developing certain types of cancers
- Improve and control blood sugar
- Lower your risk of heart diseases
- Alleviate joint pain
- Reduce cholesterol levels

So, learn to set realistic expectations when it comes to losing weight, so you can boost your sense of achievement and avoid burning out.

Focus on Your Process

Unfortunately, people do not realize that they should not only set outcome goals. It is also important for them to set process goals. An outcome goal is what you should achieve at the end of the program, which is usually the target weight. This method can affect your motivation because you do not know when you will reach that weight. You may have hit a plateau, and it will be hard for you to move past it. Outcome goals can leave you feeling overwhelmed because you can only achieve them after a period.

To avoid feeling this way, set process goals. Identify the actions you will take to reach the goal. For instance, you can say that you will work out at least four times a week while trying to lose weight. This is a process goal, and you can reward yourself once you meet it. You will also feel better about the process when you do this.

A study conducted by Pearson E S in 2012 had 126 overweight women as subjects. These women were all a part of different weight loss programs. Pearson noted that women who were a part of process-focused programs lost weight at the right pace and did not lose motivation. Unlike the women who were focused only on the outcome goals, they did not move away from their diets.

Therefore, you need to set SMART goals for yourself:

- Specific
- Measurable
- Attainable
- Realistic
- Time-based

Consider the following examples of SMART goals or process goals you should have:

- I will walk for at least 30 minutes every day for a week.
- I will limit snacking to only one day a week.
- I will not drink soda this week.

Choose a Plan that Suits Your Lifestyle

You must find a plan that is easy for you to stick to. Do not choose plans that you cannot follow easily in the future. There are a lot of diets out there, and most of these are based on calorie counting. When you create a calorie deficit in your body, it will help you lose weight. Dieting, however, especially if you constantly switch from one diet to the other, can lead to weight gain in the future. Therefore, you should focus on the type of diet you choose to follow. Never follow a diet that expects you to eliminate certain foods completely.

A study conducted by Teixiera P J et al. in 2012 concluded that people could not follow a diet or a dietary pattern if they needed to eliminate foods. When you eliminate foods from your diet, your body begins to crave them, and this will make it harder for you to stick to your diet. Work on developing a plan that works for you. Keep the following tips in mind when you prepare the plan:

- Increase your intake of fruits and vegetables
- Decrease your caloric intake
- Reduce desserts and fried food
- Reduce portion sizes
- Reduce the frequency of snacks

Maintain a Journal

It is important to monitor yourself if you want to lose weight successfully. As mentioned earlier, self-monitoring is one way to motivate yourself to stick to your diet. A study conducted by Kong A et al. in 2012 had people who were in weight loss programs as subjects. Some subjects were asked to maintain a journal, while others did not. The research team found that people who tracked their food intake were able to lose weight faster. They also found it easier to maintain their weight loss.

Having said that, it is important to make notes correctly if you choose to maintain a food journal. You need to write everything down. This means you need to include details of all your snacks, meals, and even the slice of cake you ate at work. If you want to make the process effective, note down your emotions, too. This information will help you identify any triggers causing you to binge or overeat. Use this information to learn how to cope with such situations.

You can either use an application or website to maintain a food journal. These are known to be effective.

Apps to Use as Food Journals

Food does not affect your weight alone. It also affects your health, mood, and various lifestyle factors. The following are some applications that you can use to track your intake, and it may seem like a pain to do this, especially because you may snack. It is a good habit to maintain a food journal and identify everything you consume. You need to know what you are putting into your body. This is honestly a great way for you to learn more about yourself.

Some of the best food diary applications you can use are listed below. Each of these follows a different approach, so choose the one that works best for you.

- **See How You Eat**

This app is compatible with both Android and iOS. It is a visual food diary, which means you need to take pictures of everything you eat. This is the easiest way to maintain a food journal. This application is still a work in progress, but it is great if you are only starting off with maintaining a food journal.

The objective of the application is to avoid calorie counting. Most food diary applications use calorie counting, and this is a turn-off for most people. This application does not require you to do anything more than taking a picture of the food you are eating. If you are new to this, you may forget to do this, so the application reminds you. This way, you can remember to take pictures whenever needed.

The objective is for you to take a picture of everything you send into your body, which means you need to take a picture of the glass of water you are drinking, too. You can only upload 12 pictures a day, and there are some bugs, too. The application, however, works well if you want to develop the habit of tracking your intake.

- **YouEat**

This app can also be used on both Android and iOS. This is an amazing food journal and tracker application, which expects you to chart the path of every meal you eat. You can also use this application to determine why you ate a certain meal. Using this application, you can identify the triggers that made you eat a specific type of food. You can also determine why you did not stick to your diet plan.

Let us look at how the application works. You click a picture of the food you are eating and either put it on your off-path or on-path. I am sure you know the path being referred to; on-path refers to food on your diet plan. Meanwhile, if you eat something you should not have, add it to your off-path list. When you add this to the off-path, you also need to indicate why you ate that meal. Was it because you were upset, angry, hungry, stressed, or anxious? Did you eat the food because you were craving something? It is important to add notes, so you are aware of why you behave a certain way.

If you use the application regularly and accurately, this becomes a great way for you to determine why you choose certain foods and the reason for choosing those foods. It is important to add these reasons to identify what makes you eat certain foods and why you chose to break your diet. It is this information that can help you stick to your weight loss plan. You can also use a recipe management application to track the foods you eat or if you want to learn some new recipes.

- **RiseUp**

RiseUp is an app you can use on both Android and iOS. Using this application, you can determine how certain foods affect your mood. This application understands that the food you eat affects you mentally. This is especially true if you have any disorder. The application allows you to track all the food you ate and how you felt after eating the food. You can also track how you felt before you ate the food, giving you a pattern.

RiseUp also has a meal log, which you can use to add the food you ate when you ate it, whether you ate alone or with someone else, and how you ate it. You can also add information about how you felt during your meal. The application comes with some target behaviors that you can use to determine how you act after a meal, such as binge eating or weighing yourself. The objective of this application is to help you identify any patterns about yourself.

The application reminds you to check on yourself and your emotions frequently. It also expects you to check in with yourself and understand how you think and feel. When you combine this data, you get an idea of how your food intake affects the way you behave and act.

- **Cara**

Cara is an advanced app that comes with a full-body tracker. You can download this on both iOS and Android. If you have been using food journals for quite some time, this is the application for you. Use it if you want to connect with your water and food consumption. Use the information on the application to help you connect the food you eat with different symptoms in your life. The application also tracks various factors, and you can use this information to understand your thoughts and habits easily.

Like other applications, this also requires you to add notes every time you drink or eat something. The application does not come with any drop-down menus. You need to type everything out and take a photo if you feel like it. Unlike most food applications, this tracks your water intake, as well. If you do not drink enough water, it can affect your health in various ways, so the application also reminds you to drink enough water.

The application also allows you to add other factors, such as digestion, stool, mental status, supplements, and mediation. You can also track your period frequency, workout frequency, sleep patterns, skin condition, pain, and other information. After a point, the application will identify a pattern between your food consumption and health. So, the application can tell you how eating a bar of chocolate will make you feel.

- **MyPlate**

MyPlate is a very simple app used as a calorie counting application. LiveStrong developed it, which means you have an entire community to motivate you and push you to achieve your goals. This application is like other fitness applications where you count calories, but its interface is easier to use and better when compared to other applications.

You need to key in your goals – both outcome and process goals – into the application. It also allows you to add information about your sodium and calcium intake. The next step is to log every piece of food you eat. The database has over two million foods, and you can choose the food from this list. Alternatively, you can use the barcode to identify the food you are eating. MyPlate will calculate the nutritional break-up and calories by using the information you have keyed in.

The application is like other fitness applications, such as HealthifyMe, Lifesum, and MyFitnessPal. You can use any of these applications if you prefer them to MyPlate. If you have not tried any of these applications, choose MyPlate because it is easier to start with it.

- **Celebrate**

It is hard to lose weight, so it is important to celebrate when you achieve your goals. This is the easiest way to motivate yourself to stick to the diet plan. When you accomplish a goal, you need to reward yourself. If you do not have anybody to tell this to, you can post it on a weight loss forum, community page, or social media. These are great places for you to share how you are doing. People on these platforms are willing to lend support. You will also feel better about yourself, which will motivate you.

You should also celebrate any changes in behavior; this is not only if you reach the target weight. For instance, if you walked for thirty minutes five days this week, go out with your friends or celebrate at home. Rewarding yourself is a great way to increase motivation. It is important to choose the right rewards. Do not use food as a reward because that will only throw you off your diet. Do not choose expensive items as rewards, either, as you cannot buy all of them. It is also important to never choose something insignificant because then you would not want to buy it.

Some examples of rewards are:

- Taking a cooking class
- Getting a manicure

- Buying a new running top
- Going to a movie

Find Support

You may need to find support groups or people who will support you on your journey. This is another great way to stay motivated. Speak with your close friends and family members about your plan, and ask if they can help you on your journey. Most people find it easier to lose weight when they have a partner. This way, you can work out together and encourage each other. You can also monitor what the other person is doing.

It is best to have support from your family because you all eat together. Having said that, you need someone outside of your family to support you, too. Alternatively, you can join an online support group or an offline one, depending on what works best for you. These groups are beneficial because every member of the group is willing to listen to you.

Commit to the Plan

A study conducted by Hayes S C et al. in 1985 noted that people who committed to anything publicly were more likely to stick to their plan and follow it through. When you tell people around you about your plan to lose weight, they may extend their support on social media. If you share your goals with more people, you will be held accountable. You can also invest in an exercise package or gym membership. As you made an investment, you will be more likely to follow through and meet your goals.

Ooze Positivity

If you have positive expectations, you will feel confident about yourself. You know you can achieve your goals and meet your ideal or target weight. You can use a concept called change talk to motivate you to achieve your goals. Change talk is where you make a statement about committing to changing some behaviors. You can also write down why you want to make this change and how you will make it. This means you need to talk positively about your plans to lose weight. You can also talk about the various processes you will begin and how you will commit to your goals.

Having said that, if you fantasize about your goals without actually doing anything to achieve them, you are not going to achieve your goals. This is a process called mental indulging, and it does more harm than good. You should use a process called mental contrast to change the way you behave and think about your weight loss plan. Spend some time every day to imagine how you will feel if you reach your goals. You can also spend some time imagining the different hurdles that can come your way and find a way to overcome them.

A study conducted by Benyamini Y and Raz O in 2007 had 134 students as subjects. The researchers asked some students to use mental indulging and others to use mental contrast to understand their goals. Students who used mental contrast acted faster when compared to those who did not. They reduced their caloric intake, avoided high-calorie food, and exercised often.

Based on this study, we can conclude that people who use mental contrast can better motivate and push themselves to meet their goals when compared to those who use mental indulging. Using the latter technique, you can trick your brain into believing that you have achieved your goal, and this will cause you not to do anything.

Plan for Any Setbacks and Hurdles

You are going to have regular stressors, and you need to plan for them. Work toward developing the right coping skills to ensure you stick to your plan and motivate yourself no matter what happens in your life. There will be parties, holidays, and birthdays to attend. You are also going to have stressors in your family and at work. Therefore, you need to brainstorm and find a way to overcome these stressors without breaking off from your weight loss plan. This is the only way you can motivate yourself and stay on track.

Most people cave in under stress and reach for their comfort food. This means they abandon their weight loss plan. It is important to develop the right coping skills if you want to avoid this.

A study conducted by Elfhag K and Rössner S in 2005 concluded that people could handle stress if they have the right strategies. They can use these strategies to help them lose weight easily and maintain their weight. Some means to cope with stress include:

- Go outside and get some fresh air

- Exercise

- Practice square breathing

- Ask for help

- Call a friend

- Take a bath

It is also important to plan for social events and holidays. You cannot expect never to eat out. If you are keen on maintaining your diet, choose the place when you meet your friends. If you are at a party and cannot find food you can eat, go for smaller portions, and choose healthier foods.

Learn to Forgive Yourself

Bear in mind that you are human and bound to make mistakes. You cannot expect to do everything correctly. So, do not strive for perfection. As mentioned earlier, an all-or-nothing attitude will just make it harder for you to lose weight. If you restrict yourself too much, you will cave in every time some good food comes into view. For instance, if you see your colleagues grabbing a burger and fries outside work, you will cave in and eat that with them. You will later tell yourself that you can eat a pizza for dinner because you ate a burger for lunch. Instead of doing this, you need to tell yourself to eat a healthy dinner because you had a big lunch.

Do not beat yourself up if you make a mistake. If you have self-defeating thoughts, you cannot work toward your goal. Learn to forgive yourself, and remember that a small mistake will not make it hard for you to lose weight. Simply start from where you left off.

Appreciate and Love Your Body

A study conducted by Elfhag K and Rössner S in 2005 showed that people who had body image issues could not lose weight easily. It is important to change the way you perceive yourself if you want to lose weight easily or maintain your weight loss. People who have a better view of their body can pick a diet or weight loss plan and stick to it. They also try new activities that will help them meet their goals. One of the following can help you change the way you perceive your body:

- Appreciate and understand that your body is doing a lot for you.

- Exercise.

- Get a manicure, pedicure, or massage.

- Do something you love.

- Find a group of positive people, and stick with them.

- Avoid comparing yourself with people who are thinner than you. Do not compare yourself with models because you do not know what they did to look the way they do.

- If you find something that fits and you like it, wear it.

- Say things about yourself out loud when you look at yourself in the mirror.

Choose Activities You Enjoy

Exercise is an important aspect when it comes to weight loss. It will improve your wellbeing and help you lose weight. It is best to choose an exercise or activity you love doing, especially if you have had trouble sticking to it in the past. There are different ways and types of exercise, so explore different options, and identify what works best for you.

It is also important to determine where you would like to work out. Would you prefer working out inside the house or outside? Do you want to work out in your house or at the gym? It is also important to determine if you like exercising with a group of people or exercising alone. If you need motivation, pick a group class because the people around you can motivate you. If you do not like group classes, then you can work out at home, too.

Experts recommend you listen to music when you work out because that can motivate you. People exercise for longer when they listen to music.

Choose Your Role Model

It is best to have a role model if you want to motivate yourself to lose weight. Having said that, you should choose the right role model so you can meet your expectations. If you use pictures of supermodels to motivate you, you are not doing anything good for yourself. Choose a role model with whom you can relate. Choosing a positive and relatable role model will motivate you. You may have a friend who recently lost a lot of weight, and that friend can be your role model. If you have no idea who your role model should be, read some inspirational stories and blogs to learn about people who lost weight successfully.

Nicholas Bjorn

Get a Dog

Yes! You read that right. Get yourself a dog because he can be your companion. A study conducted by Kushner R F in 2008 concluded that a dog could help you lose weight easily. If you own a dog, your physical activity increases because you have to take him for a walk frequently.

Another study conducted by Brown S G and Rhodes R E in 2006 concluded that people who owned dogs walked at least 300 minutes every week, and people who did not have dogs only walked 168 minutes.

Dogs also support you when you work out. They love it when there is any physical activity involved and may mimic you when you work out. An added bonus is that having a pet lowers blood pressure, reduces feelings of depression and loneliness, and lowers cholesterol. This means that having a dog not only makes life happier but also improves your physical and mental wellbeing.

Consult a Professional

Never hesitate to speak with a professional to help you with your plan and efforts. It is only when you are confident about your plan that you will lose weight. You can find a nutrition specialist or dietician to determine which foods you can eat. Alternatively, you can meet a physiologist if you want to learn how to exercise properly.

People often do better when they are accountable to a professional. If it is hard to motivate yourself, meet a dietician or psychologist who can motivate you. This is a great way for you to achieve your goals.

Nicholas Bjorn

Chapter 10: Morning Habits to Help You Lose Weight

Regardless of your outcome goals, it is hard for people to lose weight, especially if they hit a plateau. That said, you do not have to change your diet and lifestyle entirely if you want to lose weight. It is easy to lose weight if you make a few changes to your routine. This chapter will look at ten habits you should incorporate into your morning routine if you want to lose weight.

Eat Protein-Rich Foods for Breakfast

There is a reason why people say you should eat breakfast. It is the most important meal because your body would have been fasting all night. The food you consume for breakfast will determine the food you eat throughout the day. Your breakfast determines if you are full until lunch or need to hit the snack bar at work for something at 11 a.m.

If you eat a high-protein meal, it can reduce cravings until lunch and help you lose weight. A study conducted by Hoertel H A et al. in 2014 concluded that adolescents, especially girls, who ate a protein-rich breakfast lose weight easily because the meal curbed their cravings. Another small study conducted by Leidy J H et al. in 2014 concluded that a high-protein breakfast ensured you do not gain too much fat as you are less hungry throughout the day.

Protein can reduce the levels of the hunger hormone ghrelin in your body, and this can decrease your appetite. Another small study conducted by Blom A M W et al. in 2006 had 15 men as subjects. Some were asked to consume a protein-rich breakfast while others ate a normal meal. It was found that a high-protein breakfast was more effective in lowering the levels of ghrelin in the body. If you want to start your day on a good note, eat eggs, cottage cheese, chia seeds, nuts, and Greek yogurt.

Hydrate

This is very important to bear in mind. It is best to begin your day with one or two glasses of water. This is an easy way to make it easier to lose weight. Water can increase the rate at which your body burns calories for at least an hour. A study conducted by Boschmann M et al. in 2003 concluded that drinking at least 500 ml of water every day when you wake up increases your metabolic rate by 30%. They further noted that people who drank water immediately after they woke up reduced their caloric intake by 13%.

Another study conducted by Stookey D J et al. in 2008 used overweight women as subjects. The women were asked to increase their water intake by one liter every day, and they lose at least 4 pounds more than people who did not increase their water intake. They were not asked to make any changes to their diet or exercise more.

When you drink water, it reduces your food intake and appetite. Research shows that it is best to drink at least 1.5 liters of water every day if you want to lose weight. It is best to start with a glass of water every morning and hydrate yourself throughout the day if you want to lose weight without making too much of an effort.

Measure Yourself

Another good thing to do is to measure your weight every morning. This is an effective way to motivate yourself. You can also improve your control and avoid eating foods that you should not. Several studies and research show that people lose weight faster when they weigh themselves every morning. A study conducted by Steinberg M D et al. in 2015 used 47 adults as subjects. The researchers noted that people who weighed themselves regularly for over six months lost weight faster than those who did not weigh themselves enough.

Another study conducted by VanWormer J V et al. in 2012 reported that adults who weighed themselves every morning lost 10 pounds in two years while those who did not gained weight. The latter only weighed themselves once a month. When you weigh yourself regularly, you will develop healthy behaviors and habits to help you lose weight. Another study was conducted by Butryn M L et al. (2007) on a large group of adults. Some adults were asked to weigh themselves regularly, while others were asked to stop weighing themselves. At the end of the study, the researchers concluded that the latter group did not have self-discipline and increased their caloric intake.

It is best to weigh yourself when you wake up, and you need to do this immediately after you use the bathroom and before you drink or eat anything. It is also important to understand that your weight will fluctuate regularly, and this is because of various factors. Therefore, you need to focus on your outcome and look for the trends. Do not worry about the changes that happen regularly.

Get Some Sunlight

Experts recommend you open the curtains every morning for sunlight. This is a great way to kick-start your metabolism. All you need to do is sit under the sun for a few minutes. A study conducted by Reid K J et al. in 2014 concluded that even limited exposure to the sun during the day could help you lose weight. Experts also believe that ultraviolet radiation can control or suppress weight gain, but further research is needed to confirm the same.

When you expose yourself to enough sunlight every day, you can meet your daily requirement for vitamin D. Research shows that your consumption of vitamin D directly impacts your weight. It can prevent weight gain, thereby helping you maintain your weight.

Mason C et al. conducted a study in 2014 where 218 obese and overweight women were the subjects. These women were either given a placebo or a vitamin D supplement for a year. Based on their findings, the researchers concluded that women who met their daily vitamin D requirement lost 7 pounds more than women who did not meet the requirement.

Another study conducted by LeBlanc E S et al. in 2012 had 4,659 older women as subjects and tracked them for four years. They found that people with more vitamin D in their bodies did not gain too much weight.

Your skin type determines the time you need to spend under the sun. Having said that, it is a good idea to let some sunlight into your house or sit outside for a few minutes every day.

Be Mindful

Mindfulness is a technique used to stay in the present and focus on what is happening around you. It is about being aware of your feelings and thoughts. This technique can promote healthy eating habits and aid in weight loss. For instance, an analysis performed by Carrière K et al. in 2018 showed that mindfulness-based methods or techniques helped people stop eating too much food. They also noted that incorporating mindfulness into a weight loss program could increase the chances of losing weight by 68%.

It is easy to practice mindfulness. If you want to start, all you need to do is spend a few minutes every morning to connect with your senses and learn to focus on the present.

Exercise

Exercising in the morning is the best way for you to lose weight. Alizadeh A et al. conducted a study in 2015 with a group of 50 obese women as subjects. These women were asked to perform different aerobic exercises at different times of the day. There were no differences identified between the food cravings of women who exercised in the afternoon when compared to the food cravings of women who exercised in the morning. However, the research team noted that women who exercised in the morning were not as hungry as women who exercised at a later part of the day.

When you exercise in the morning, you can maintain your blood sugar levels, thus reducing any hunger pangs or cravings. A study conducted by Gomez A M et al. in 2015 concluded that people who have type 1 diabetes have less trouble with blood sugar control during the day if they work out in the morning. These studies focused only on certain populations and did not discuss causation. Further research is needed to determine when people should exercise.

Change Your Mode of Transport

It is easy to drive to work or anywhere else you may need to go. This is not great for your visceral or abdominal fat. Research shows that using public transportation, walking, and biking is probably the best way to lose weight and reduce the risk of gaining weight. A study conducted by Sugiyama T et al. in 2013 followed 822 subjects for a period of four years. The research team found that people who often traveled by car were more obese compared to those who did not.

Another study conducted by Flint E et al. in 2014 followed a group of 15,777 people and concluded that using public or active methods of transport, such as biking or walking, helped to lower body fat percentage and body mass index when compared to using cars. Work on changing your mode of transport at least twice or thrice a week.

Focus on Your Intake

I know you know this by now, but this is an important point to bear in mind. It is only when you track your intake that you can lose weight easily. When you focus on the foods you eat, you learn to hold yourself accountable. Research shows that tracking your food helps you lose weight easily. You know exactly what you are putting into your body and know what needs to be done to lose weight.

A study conducted by Anton D S et al. in 2012 concluded that people who used a system to track their food intake and monitor their exercise and diet lost weight faster than the people who did not track this information. Another study conducted by Peterson D N et al. in 2015 used 220 overweight and obese women as subjects. The research team concluded that consistent and frequent use of self-monitoring applications and tools helped these women lose weight easily.

You can use an application or even maintain a diary to list the foods you drink and eat.

Nicholas Bjorn

Chapter 11: Small Lifestyle Changes to Lose Weight

It may feel at times that you can lose weight only when you starve or deprive your body of calories, but this is not the case. The author of "Small Steps to Slim," Ashvini Mashru, says, "Healthy, sustainable weight loss is best achieved through small changes to your existing lifestyle." She reminds everybody that weight loss is a process. It is not a sprint, and you cannot lose weight in five days.

It is easier to adopt fad diets as you can drop a size in less than a week, but you are not going to stick to these diets in the long run. The weight will definitely drop quickly, but you will gain all the lost weight and more in a very short time if you do not take care of yourself. This chapter has some tips you can use to ensure you healthily lose weight. These are small lifestyle changes you can make to ensure you maintain or improve your health despite losing weight.

Focus on the Portions

According to Mashru, most Americans do not stick to their portion sizes. They eat twice the amount they should. Restaurants serve large portions of food, which will train your brain into thinking this is the amount of food you need to eat. If you want to understand your portions better, you should check the nutritional labels and understand the information given on those labels.

Pause Between Bites

You must chew slowly, as this is a simple way to lower your caloric intake. If you take time to chew instead of swallowing your food quickly, your body will feel full faster. Experts believe it takes your body only 20 minutes to feel full and for this feeling to reach your brain. If you eat slowly, you can relish the meal and eat less than you used to.

Prepare Your Lunch

When you prepare your lunch, you can save a lot of money, ensuring you are aware of what you are consuming. If you work from home, you can walk up to the fridge, pick up your box of food, and heat it up in the oven. Do not skip your meal. You may lose weight faster if you deprive your body of calories, but this only means you will overdo it later during the day or week.

Focus While Eating

If there is a lot of work to do or your friend has sent you a reel on Instagram, you may want to eat quickly to get to your laptop or phone. When you are distracted while you eat, you tend to eat more than you should. Distractions can force you to eat more throughout the day.

Snack Smartly

If you are trying to lose weight, you need to snack smartly. Snacking is helpful as long as you check what you eat. You may consume more than what you should when you snack because you do not know the number of nutrients you consume. This is a simple issue to fix because you can pre-pack your snacks and portion them according to your caloric intake. Another problem with snacking is that you may eat something throughout the day without realizing what it is that you are doing. It is important to focus on your goal and manage your intake.

Sleep Well

I am sure you want to catch up on episodes of *Friends* or watch the movie *Without Remorse*. This does not mean you do not sleep enough. It is important to sleep well and get enough rest if you want to lose weight. The appetite hormones leptin and ghrelin are kept in check if you sleep enough. If you do not sleep enough, you will have an imbalance in your body, increasing your appetite. Aim to sleep for at least 7 hours every night.

Healthy Eating at All Times

Your weekend cannot be your cheat day. You cannot eat whatever you want because it is the weekend. If you do this regularly, you will not lose weight the way you hoped you would. Eating poorly on weekends and not exercising is like taking 12 days off in a month, and this is not going to help with weight loss. Do not let the days of the week change the way you eat or behave. Focus on your healthy lifestyle, and ensure you sustain yourself throughout the week.

Use Small Plates

How does the same quantity of food look to you on a small plate when compared to a large plate? Your eyes will convince you that the smaller plate has more food. This is because of the Delboeuf illusion, which shows that empty space around anything will make it seem a little smaller. You may not be eating too much, but if you cut back on the space you have on your plate, you can convince your brain that you have eaten enough food. If you do the opposite, your brain may push you into thinking you are hungry, and this will only make you eat more.

Avoid Family-Style Eating

When you eat with your family, your table is filled with dishes with delicious food. You may mindlessly fill your plate with more food in such situations because everybody is eating, and the food is right there. If it is possible, you should avoid cooking too much food. Limit the quantity of food on your table. This does not mean you cannot take seconds, but it does mean you need to check if you are hungry before you go in for the second helping.

Do Not Face the Buffet

If the food in the restaurant is in your line of sight, you are going to feel terrible about missing some food. You may want to get your money's worth when you go to a restaurant. Instead of eating what is on your plate while looking at what you can eat next, focus only on what is on your plate. The buffet is not going anywhere, so you can eat more food if you want to.

Eat Enough Vegetables

When you follow a diet, you need to add things to your diet instead of removing them. This is a healthy way to look at a diet. If you do not consume any food you want to eat, you will binge on it, and this will only throw you off your plan. Instead of removing food from your diet, add more vegetables to your plate gradually. This will increase your chances of losing weight. Vegetables are rich in nutrients and also keep your body energized and healthy. They satiate your hunger and keep cravings at bay. If you want to avoid hating vegetables, start off small. Add one cup of vegetables to your meal for a week, and slowly increase the quantity when you get used to them.

Nicholas Bjorn

Chapter 12: How to Create a Customized Diet Plan to Help You Lose Weight

If you want to lose weight healthily, you need to create a diet plan that works best. You must ensure your body receives the required calories and nutrients to sustain itself throughout the day, especially if you work out. It is important to maintain this balance if you want to get rid of fat and lose weight.

Your diet plan is successful if you consume the required nutrients, especially protein, to ensure your body builds muscle and maintains your energy. To do this, you need to understand your body and develop a plan that suits your needs. Use the steps in this chapter to develop a weight loss plan structured to your goals, habits, and lifestyle.

Step One: Do Not Use Calorie-Counting Diets

Most diet plans begin with setting a daily calorie limit. If you follow these diets, you need to reduce your consumption of any food you eat so that you fall within this limit. You need to eat healthy foods, so your body thrives. Unfortunately, this theory is what keeps dieters from sticking to their meal plans. They fail even before they start the diet. You need to look at different approaches to count your caloric intake.

Do you know why it is wrong to count your caloric intake every day?

- Bear in mind that every food you eat has a different number of calories. Unless you eat the same food every day, you cannot track your consumption easily. You would need to put in a lot of work, and this will throw you off

- Dieters cannot follow their diet when they go out with their friends or are on vacation. There are also other reasons why people cannot stick to their diet, one of which is that they cannot stick to their daily caloric count.

- To avoid temptation, some people designate some days as cheat days when they could eat everything they want to without worrying about their caloric intake. This is why some people do not lose weight even when they follow a low-calorie diet, especially as they over-indulge on one day.

- If you count your caloric intake regularly, you will eat less. However, most dieters choose to stay below the required caloric number, and because they miss too many calories regularly, they experience some negative effects

The objective should not be to set the number of calories you consume per day but rather to identify a plan that covers your necessities. Ensure you consume the required nutrients if you want to lead a healthy lifestyle. This is a good approach to follow when you want to lose weight. It is not restrictive and gives you enough freedom to eat the food you love in moderation.

Bear in mind that the nutritional needs of your friends and family are different from yours. These needs are based on your activity levels, weight, height, age, and medical needs. If you set the right guidelines and goals for yourself, you can eat different foods that will help you reach your goals. These goals enable you to focus on your intake of carbs, protein, minerals, vitamins, and fats. It is important to balance these nutrients to ensure your body has all the nutrition it needs.

Step Two: Calculating Your Macros

It is important to understand that dieting does not mean you control your food intake alone. Your body needs to get the right nutrition to grow muscle, burn fat, and provide enough energy to sustain you throughout the day. Your body uses macronutrients, such as carbohydrates, protein, and fat, to complete these tasks. These macronutrients constitute a major chunk of your caloric intake.

- **Carbohydrates**

Both complex and simple carbohydrates are sugar chains broken down by your body to provide energy to your organs and muscles.

- **Fats**

If you consume too many calories, your body stores them in fat cells and uses them in case of an emergency. If there are no carbohydrates that your body can burn, it will use these fat cells to produce energy. This energy is used by your body to perform hormonal and neural functions.

- **Proteins**

Proteins are known as the powerhouse macros because they provide your body with the energy it needs to grow and repair tissues.

It is important to balance these nutrients if you want to build a body that is not exhausted all the time. These nutrients also ensure you do not feel deprived of energy. A rule of thumb is that you need to divide your caloric intake as follows: 25% carbohydrates, 35% healthy fat, and 40% protein. You can speak with your nutritionist or doctor if you need a better measurement.

Step Three: Find Foods That Suit You

When you are aware of the quantity you need to eat, take some time to identify which foods fall into this category. Identify the foods you can regularly consume when you change your eating patterns. This is an effective way to lose weight because you only include foods in the diet if you can eat them. If you do not enjoy the food, you will not stick to your plan. Having said that, you need to make an effort to identify new options for your plan. Most dieters choose a weight loss program because they follow diets that limit their food intake and calories. It is essential to add more nutritional options and foods to your diet to create a long-term plan.

Make a list of all ingredients and foods you can eat. If you love something, add that to the list, too. When you begin your diet, you can add new fruits, grains, or vegetables to your plan each week. Experts recommend you include some information about the macronutrients in the foods you consume as this will help you determine whether you will enjoy your meals.

Step Four: Find Every Recipe You Can

You are now aware of the quantity of food you can eat and what you should eat. So, begin collecting a few recipes that include your preferred ingredients. Read the recipes, and understand them fully. The micronutrient content is dependent on the way you cook your food.

If you do not want weight loss to become boring, you should collect enough recipes. If you lose interest in your current menu, switch it up with other recipes. There are many reasons why people do not meet their target weight, and one of the most important ones is getting bored with the current meal plan. If you have variety, you will enjoy your meals and look forward to eating something new. You have numerous resources online, so use them to your benefit.

If you perform enough research, you can tweak and tailor any recipe you love to suit your needs. If you love pastries and cakes, find a recipe that falls within your calorie range. You do not have to quit eating foods you love because you are on a diet. You should only swap some ingredients or reduce the quantity of every ingredient you use. If you are worried about giving up fries, you can find a recipe that uses an oven to create a crispy outer covering.

If you lead a stressful life, compile a list of restaurants that serve food that meets your nutrient requirements. You can also meet the staff and ask for additional information if you want. You can use the information you have to identify a list of restaurants you can visit within your budget.

Step Five: Set a Schedule

It is important to determine when you eat, as this is as important as choosing what to eat. Your body constantly works and has a cycle, which affects your metabolism. There is a cycle that specifically works on your metabolism, and medical conditions can change the way that cycle works. This means you might not lose as much weight as you once hoped.

A diet plan includes three meals for most people, but this does not always work, especially for those who want to cut back on their caloric intake. It is best to have meals at regular intervals. Do not give your body too much of a gap between each meal during the day. You can give yourself a three-hour window between each meal. This will keep your hunger at bay and prevent you from eating unhealthy food. The following are some ways to help you develop a plan:

- Eat a heavy dinner if you want to avoid snacking at night

- Eat a high-protein breakfast an hour after you wake up

- Stick to the meal plan

If you have any glucose conditions or diabetes, speak with a dietician or nutritionist to know what you should eat. Ensure you develop a plan that works best for your body.

Step Six: Track, Adjust, and Analyze

As mentioned earlier, maintaining a food journal can go a long way. You can keep track of your meal plan and maintain a record of the food you eat. This gives you a chance to understand your eating habits and determine whether your plan works for you. It is important to adjust your plan when you need to if you want to lose or maintain weight. Do not worry about making changes to your plan if you do not achieve your required results.

Nicholas Bjorn

Chapter 13: How to Manage Your Weight Loss

You may have lost a lot of weight throughout your plan and do not want that number to go up. It seems inevitable that you will gain the weight back, but this does not have to be the case if you take care of yourself. An analysis conducted by the National Weight Control Registry showed that it is easy for people to maintain their weight in the long term. The following are some tips you can use to keep losing weight and keep that weight off the scale.

Build Lean Muscle

It is important to maintain your metabolism when you lose weight. You can do this by building lean muscle. Bear in mind that your body has a higher metabolic rate when you have more muscle than fat. If you do not use weights, it is best to add some resistance to your exercise routine now. Doing this will help you increase the weight you work with and challenge yourself.

Eat More Filling Foods

You are bound to feel hungry, but it is important to find a way to keep yourself from eating too much. As mentioned earlier, you can only avoid snacking and binging if you eat full meals. When you increase your fiber and nutrient intake, your hunger will be satiated, and you will not snack every chance you get.

Curb Temptation

Yes, you are not supposed to eat too much of some type of food. This does not mean you should never eat them. You are allowed to give yourself a break every now and then, but it is important never to do it when you are tempted. You can control your weight if you do not give in to your cravings and temptations. It is easy to avoid these temptations by planning your meals ahead, removing any comfort foods or weaknesses from the pantry, and eating out less than you used to.

Count Your Calories

According to the University of Pittsburgh, people lose weight and maintain their weight easily if they watch their caloric intake. You can use a food journal application and make notes about all your meals throughout the day. This helps you track your caloric intake. People are successful at maintaining their weight if they count their calories and limit their intake of fat.

Meal Plans

A weight maintenance diet is like a weight loss diet because you need to plan your meals. If you have a plan ready, it is easy for you to stick to it. Your weight loss plan will have fewer calories when compared to your maintenance plan, but this will keep you on track.

Increase Your Activity Time

Experts recommend that people should exercise for at least 30 minutes every day for at least five days a week. This is only when it comes to losing weight. If you want to maintain your weight, you need to exercise more than you used to. You can walk or perform any activity you like for at least 50 minutes every day if you want to lose weight. You can burn more calories than before and maintain your weight.

Watch Your Portion Sizes

The Centers for Disease Control and Prevention (CDC) conducted a study with 4000 adults as the participants. The research team noted that people who measured their fat and protein intake successfully maintained their weight. This does not mean you have to measure everything you eat, but you should do this at home, so you know how to measure portion sizes if you eat out. It is important to do this so you do not overeat or eat foods that do not help you maintain your weight.

Regular Weighing

It is important to weigh yourself regularly. We have discussed this in detail earlier in the book. If you weigh yourself daily, you will succeed at losing weight and maintaining it. It can be discouraging to weigh yourself regularly if you follow a diet, but this is a great way to maintain your weight.

Eat Dairy

When you eat enough dairy products, specifically low-fat products, you can reduce your hunger pangs. If you crave something sweet, grab a cup of yogurt, and top it with berries. The extra calcium can also improve your bone health, and this is especially important for women.

Use Your Plate as Your Guide

If you cannot measure portions or calculate your caloric intake correctly, use a cup or plate method. This way, you can control your intake. This is a tip commonly used by people on a diet, but it is a great way for you to maintain your weight as well. When you use this method, you need to cover half your plate with vegetables and divide the other half between whole grains and protein. If you do want another helping, swap the whole grains and protein for dairy and fruit.

Stop Watching too much TV

You can maintain your weight easily if you focus on what you are eating. You need to spend time chewing your vegetables and not worrying about why a character on a show wanted revenge.

Chapter 14: Final Push – 21 More Ways to Remain Motivated

This final chapter is just one more set of motivations – things that should give you the push you need to continue on your journey. It will be a long journey, make no mistake about it, but if you are fully prepared mentally, then there will not be a challenge that you cannot overcome.

Think of motivation as being something like the gas you put in your car – the tank doesn't need to be completely full for it to run, but it mustn't be allowed to run empty. Don't ever waste precious time on trying to keep your motivation levels at the maximum because that in itself will wear you down. Motivation has its own natural rhythm – if your motivation levels drop, don't see it as a failure because it isn't.

1. Give it a rest

If your motivation levels start to drop off, take a break from your diet or your fitness regime – just for a period of one to three days, no more. The biggest problem with motivation is that, the more you try catching it, the more elusive it is going to become, so let the natural motivation rhythm run its course. By doing this and by having a plan of habit-changing skills drawn up, you will find it much easier to stay on track, and your motivation levels will simply follow their own natural rhythm

2. Question yourself

When you need a bit of quick inspiration and a bit of a reminder about why you are doing this, ask yourself these questions. Answering them honestly can often be just the boost that you need to carry on:

- What will I look like in six months or a year if I stop my diet?

- How will I feel in six months or a year if I stop my diet?

- What will my health be like if I stop my diet?

- What effect will it have on the people around me – my family, my friends, and myself – if I stop my diet?

Be honest in your answers; if you are not, the only person you are kidding is you.

3. Clean your closet out

If you are finding it tough to stick to your intention to lose weight and get fit, turn to another area of your life. Clean your closet out. Sort out your clothes into those that you will never ever wear again, those that are a size (or two) too small, and those that you wear now. Ditch the clothes you will not wear again, give them to charity, and then look at what is left. Do you want to get into those smaller clothes again or not? Another thing you could do is focus your attention on paying off your debts. The idea is to learn how to stick to a commitment that you have made; if you can do that in one area of your life, you can do it in another, and the sight of those too-small clothes should be just enough motivation to kick you back into gear.

Weight Loss Motivation

4. Don't keep looking at pictures of models who are super skinny

While it might seem like great inspiration to have pictures of super-skinny models posted everywhere, recent studies have shown that, in fact, the opposite is true. The research involved a group of women who wanted to drop some weight who divided into two groups. Each group was given a food journal to complete – group one had pictures of skinny models on the pages, and group two had a neutral images on theirs. Group two – those with the neutral images – lost weight, whereas the group that had the pictures of the models actually gained weight.

Looking at pictures of these super-thin women is very discouraging for one simple reason – you are creating self-standards that are simply not realistic. If you spend your time looking at a picture of a much thinner woman while you are eating, you are more likely to feel that there is no way on earth you can reach that weight or look, so there isn't any point in trying. Instead of those pictures, look at pictures of you when you were at a good weight and were healthy.

5. Focus on feeling

So many of people focus our entire attention on what number the scale is on and what number they want to reach, or maybe even on the workouts that they have to do to get to that number. That is quite possibly one of the quickest ways to kill off your motivation. Try focusing on something else – how do you feel after you have eaten a wonderful healthy meal or after you finished that last workout? How do you feel when you wake up in the mornings now? Motivation doesn't always have to come first – sometimes, the activity or the feeling you get from that activity can be enough to give you the motivation you need to carry on. Focus on how you are feeling when you finish a run, how many calories you have just burned off, and how good you feel deep inside.

6. Have a "business" plan

All ventures need some kind of plan, especially if they are to be successful. That plan must lay out what the mission or goal is and how you are going to get there. The same goes for when you are looking to lose weight. If you don't have that plan, you don't have the first idea on where you should be starting, where you are heading, or even how you are going to get there.

Your weight loss goal is your business objective. One you know what it is you want to achieve and when you want to achieve it by, then and only then can you begin to work out how you are going to get there. Make sure that your goals are specific and reasonable. It's no good setting goals that are simply not attainable; that's the first step towards failure. Also, don't include any strategies that just won't work, simply because you feel you should.

7. Set a halfway marker

While it is a great idea to give yourself a reward for reaching your goals, it can sometimes take months, even years, to get to a specific point. If you are waiting that long for your rewards, the wind is going to be knocked right out of your sails before you even get your end goal in sight. Instead of waiting to pass the checkered flag at the end, plan a few small treats along the way and something big for the halfway point – something like that cruise you always wanted to do. If you have something like that to look forward to, you are less likely to give up when the going gets tough. I can tell you that it's around that mid-point that things will start to get tough.

8. Act "as if"

Don't wait until you've got that bikini body to take your holiday, go and visit an old friend, or even take up that dance class you've been dreaming of. Do it now; live your life, and enjoy it. Act as though you are already at the weight you want to be at. Think about how you would feel, how you would eat and drink, and what your day would look like. What are you not doing until you reach that weight? Do it now, and move your mind out of punishment mode and into a rewarding mode – one that makes you want to stick at it.

9. Put your motivation on the mirror

I mentioned putting inspirational quotes on your mirror earlier, but you could also go down the route of pinning a photo of you at your best on there or a pair of skinny jeans that you WILL get back into. Pick a special outfit – something that you are really looking forward to putting on – and hang it by your mirror. See yourself wearing it; think about how good it is going to feel to get into it. As it is a photo of you or an item of your clothing, it is a much more realistic goal than pinning those pictures of super-skinny models up.

10. Tough love

Okay, it can be very motivating to see yourself wearing that special outfit, but some people find it even more inspiring and more motivating to imagine how they would be if they did not lose the weight. Ask yourself what life will be like for you in 10 or 20 years if you don't change the path you are travelling. Try to visualize the weight you will be at and the level of fitness you might or might not have, as the case may be. Try to imagine the health conditions that you could have as a result of not making those changes now. Be very honest with yourself here – it's all too easy to say that it'll never happen to you and that everything is just fine. It isn't, or you wouldn't have opted to start your weight loss journey in the first place.

11. Be Competitive

When it comes to shedding ponds, even a small amount of competition can take you a long way. Recent studies have shown that taking part in team-based competitions for losing weight can result in you dropping up to 20% more weight than you would if you were to do it alone. Team captains were shown to lose even more weight than the members of their teams, probably because of the involvement and position they hold in the team. So, if you really want to boost your success rate, get a team together, and head for victory.

12. Why are you really exercising?

The key to maintaining motivation is focusing on what really motivates you to do something. If your family is your inspiration, think about how your diet and exercise plan is going to help you to be around longer for your kids. Then, get your family involved in your plan. Get your partner to come to the gym with you, play physical games with the kids, and get together at the weekend and cook a whole bunch of healthy meals for the week ahead. If you are going to change the patterns of your behavior, you have first got to recognize the patterns and understand why they exist. Once you have done that, your motivation levels can be redirected towards the right areas, and your goal will suddenly seem far more achievable and realistic.

13. A photo a day

A picture really is worth a thousand words sometimes, and in today's age of digital technology and smartphones, it is much easier than it has ever been to build up your own library for personal motivation. Track your progress with a photo app, like Instagram. Post a photo a day, and document all those changes that you probably would not notice otherwise and that scale doesn't always show. You might just be surprised at what you can see in a photo that you didn't see in the mirror.

14. Shut your inner-critic up

We all have that inner critic – the one that criticizes us all the time. That is our bad habit – a way of using self-criticism as a way of trying to motivate ourselves. I've got news for you: It doesn't work. Not only will it not give you any motivation, but it is actually likely to put a serious kink in your efforts as well. When you criticize yourself, what you are doing is engaging a certain part of the brain – the bit that monitors and controls your fight or flight reflex. The result is an increase in the secretion of cortisol, which is a stress hormone, and that, in turn, makes you want foods that are fatty and sweet – comfort foods.

Next time you find yourself in self-critical mode, put your hand over your heart. Hold it there, and breathe in deeply a few times. This changes the psychological state that your mind is in and shuts the negativity down.

15. Have health all around you

Change your home to reflect the new you – the lighter, healthier you. Stock up your fridge with healthy foods, and place prepped foods in clear containers so you can see them. Fill up bowls with fresh fruit, and leave them on the counters. Put all your workout shoes on a nice shoe rack, on display by the front door. Don't leave dirty laundry on your exercise equipment. There is so much you can do to reflect what you want to be that will make it a whole lot easier to follow your plan and stick to it.

16. Use your smartphone

These days, the mobile app stores are packed full of weight loss apps, carb counters, calorie counters, and recipe apps – you name it, and it's there. Picking the right ones to use can mean that you motivation is no more than one tap away. Use the apps to come up with ideas for healthy nutritional meals, to give you the boost you need to get on the way to the gym, or to get some ideas on new exercises. There are plenty to choose from, and you will surely find something that will keep you on the go and moving forward.

17. Write down your personal reasons for losing weight

While we all want to look great in that new outfit or look fit and toned on the beach, sometimes, that just isn't enough motivation to keep you going. Sit down, and write a list of every single reason why you should lose weight. Write down all the things that would be better about you and your life if you weighed less. Perhaps it's feeling a lot healthier, having more confidence, shopping for funky new clothes, or just being able to keep up with your kids – all the things that would be so much easier to do if you just dropped those pounds. Keep your list on hand, and look at it all the time. Remind yourself of why you are doing this and why it's worth sticking to.

18. Recruit some gift givers

It is nice to reward yourself along the way – or at least the thought of it is. Sometimes, the theory is much easier than the practice, and you often become so busy that you simply don't have time to stop and reward yourself. Instead, get your friends involved. Give a few of them $20 to go and buy you a surprise, wrap it up, and give it you. Set the gift giving at certain points – say one gift for every 10 lbs. lost. That is a great way to keep yourself motivated and a nice surprise to look forward to at certain milestones.

19. Set goals that don't rely on the scales

You can do everything right, but sometimes, those scales will just not move, and the weight just does not seem to be shifting as quickly as you would like. Never let that get to you or discourage you. Set other goals – not just a number on the scale. Set little in-between goals, like working out for an extra 10 or 20 minutes a week, running just that bit further, and sticking to your schedule like glue. Then, reward yourself for all of these little goals.

Set goals like staying inside of your calorie range for so many days at a time, for dinking 64 ounces of water a day, or packing up your lunch every day so you don't get tempted by forbidden foods. Celebrating each new goal is a great way to keep your motivation in gear. You may be surprised at how much quicker the weight seems to come off. Do not focus on a number; focus on life instead.

20. Face your fears

Sometimes, it isn't a lack of motivation that gets in your way; it's your fears or your beliefs that are holding you back. Maybe you have been trying to lose weight by exercising but find yourself taking a different route that doesn't go past the gym or not going out for that walk. Ask yourself why this is. Is it because you simply don't want to do the exercise? Is it because you are embarrassed by how you look in your running gear? To get round this, list some alternatives that will keep you on the move, such as doing fitness DVDs at home instead.

21. Cultivate some compassion

If you get to a stage where you feel totally uninspired or are having a down period about what your body looks like, move your focus elsewhere – to some self-appreciation. Don't beat yourself up if you did not reach your goal this week, and instead, be grateful for the fact that you are healthy and that your body can move and do many things for you. Move from thinking about you look to how you feel and function, cultivating a little compassion and gratitude for the body that got you through another week.

Nicholas Bjorn

Conclusion

Thank you again for purchasing this book!

I hope this book was able to help you to develop a plan to lose weight and maintain your motivation while you work towards your goals.

The next step is to put your plan into action. You can go back to this book anytime you feel down. In times when your motivation dips, you should read the strategies suggested in this book again. This will help you find the best one that is applicable to your situation.

One quote that I did not mention above and one that is very true is "weight loss is NOT a physical challenge; it's a mental one." The determination that you need to succeed and your motivation, inspiration, positivity, strength, enthusiasm, willpower, encouragement, desire, and pride are all determining factors in the success of your weight loss journey, and they all come from within your mind.

Many people believe that losing weight is purely physical, but when you begin to see it as a mental challenge, you will have more chance of success, and you will find it easier to move through that journey. If your mind isn't in gear before you start – if you haven't mentally prepared yourself – it just isn't going to happen.

You must be prepared to do whatever it takes. If you're not, then you're not going anywhere. The only person who can truly motivate you is you. You are the only one who can give yourself the kick you need to carry on, and you are the only one who can truly encourage and cheer yourself as you overcome obstacle after obstacle.

Be warned that the journey to losing weight is not an easy one, and you have to be mentally prepared to do it. Don't expect results overnight because you will be disappointed. It took a long time to add that extra weight to your body, and it's going to take a long while to shift it safely.

Yes, there are plenty of crash diets you can do that will get rid of pounds of fat in a week, but think about this carefully – just how sustainable is that diet? It isn't – I can tell you that now, for free. As soon as you start finding a particular diet difficult to do, you will stop doing it, and you will go straight back to your old ways. Not only will you gain back the weight you lost, but you will most likely gain back a few more pounds as well.

So, learn to take it slow, and trust the process. Your weight loss plan is not a sprint but a marathon. Trust yourself, and focus on doing things that make you happy. Keep yourself active, and eat the right foods so your energy levels do not dip. Use the different applications mentioned in this book to keep yourself on track. Lastly, do not punish yourself for making a mistake. You would not be human if you did not. If you fall off the wagon, get up, brush yourself off, and start again.

If you enjoyed this book, then I'd like to ask you for a favor – would you be kind enough to leave a review for this book on Amazon? It'd be greatly appreciated!

Thank you, and good luck!

Weight Loss Motivation

FREE E-BOOKS SENT WEEKLY

Join North Star Readers Book Club
And Get Exclusive Access To The Latest Kindle Books in
Health, Fitness, Weight Loss and Much More...

TO GET YOU STARTED HERE IS YOUR FREE E-BOOK:

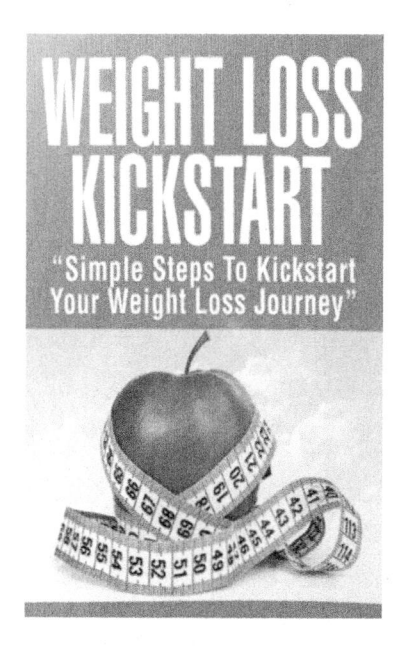

Visit to Sign Up Today!
www.northstarreaders.com/weight-loss-kick-start

Nicholas Bjorn

Resources

https://www.nhs.uk/live-well/healthy-weight/12-tips-to-help-you-lose-weight/

https://www.webmd.com/diet/obesity/features/7-ways-get-your-diet-off-good-start#3

https://www.healthline.com/nutrition/weight-loss-motivation-tips#TOC_TITLE_HDR_18

https://www.shape.com/weight-loss/tips-plans/22-ways-stay-motivated-lose-weight

https://www.healthline.com/nutrition/weight-loss-morning-habits#TOC_TITLE_HDR_11

https://www.self.com/story/small-lifestyle-habits-help-lose-weight

https://denverweightlossclinic.com/6-steps-to-creating-a-customized-diet-plan-for-weight-loss/

https://www.everydayhealth.com/weight/weight-management.aspx

https://pubmed.ncbi.nlm.nih.gov/16339128/

https://pubmed.ncbi.nlm.nih.gov/21852063/

https://www.ncbi.nlm.nih.gov/pmc/articles/PMC3312817/

https://pubmed.ncbi.nlm.nih.gov/22795495/

Nicholas Bjorn

https://www.makeuseof.com/tag/food-diary-apps/

https://www.ncbi.nlm.nih.gov/pmc/articles/PMC1308011/

https://onlinelibrary.wiley.com/doi/full/10.1111/j.1559-1816.2007.00189.x

https://pubmed.ncbi.nlm.nih.gov/15655039/

https://pubmed.ncbi.nlm.nih.gov/15655039/

https://www.researchgate.net/publication/244890224_Companion_Dogs_as_Weight_Loss_Partners

https://pubmed.ncbi.nlm.nih.gov/16459211/

https://pubmed.ncbi.nlm.nih.gov/25098557/

https://pubmed.ncbi.nlm.nih.gov/26239831/

https://pubmed.ncbi.nlm.nih.gov/16469977/

https://pubmed.ncbi.nlm.nih.gov/14671205/

https://pubmed.ncbi.nlm.nih.gov/18787524/

https://pubmed.ncbi.nlm.nih.gov/25683820/

https://pubmed.ncbi.nlm.nih.gov/21732212/

https://pubmed.ncbi.nlm.nih.gov/25555390/

https://www.ncbi.nlm.nih.gov/pmc/articles/PMC4592764/

https://pubmed.ncbi.nlm.nih.gov/29076610/

https://www.ncbi.nlm.nih.gov/pmc/articles/PMC4138353/

https://pubmed.ncbi.nlm.nih.gov/23332335/

https://www.ncbi.nlm.nih.gov/pmc/articles/PMC4149603/

https://pubmed.ncbi.nlm.nih.gov/23063049/

https://www.ncbi.nlm.nih.gov/pmc/articles/PMC3466912/

https://pubmed.ncbi.nlm.nih.gov/24622804/

https://www.ncbi.nlm.nih.gov/pmc/articles/PMC3973603/

https://pubmed.ncbi.nlm.nih.gov/18198319/

GOOD NUTRITION IS IMPORTANT – THIS IS A FACT.

BUT HOW DO YOU REALLY GET STARTED TO ACHIEVING IT? PEOPLE SAY IT BEGINS WITH A BALANCED DIET, BUT HOW EXACTLY DO YOU ACHIEVE THAT BALANCE?

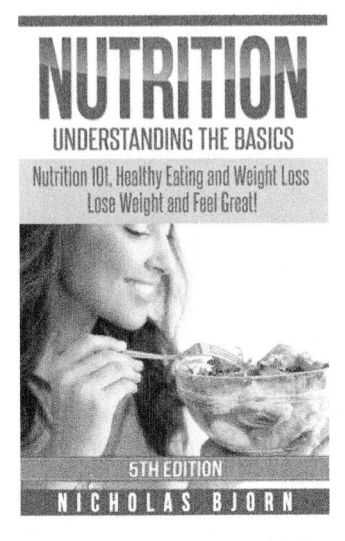

If you are lost in the world of calories and kilojoules, this book is the perfect reference to help you! The contents of this book will help you focus on what's important while getting rid of all the unnecessary fluff about dieting and healthy living that are just bound to confuse you.

Here is what this book has in store for you:
- Nutrition defined and simplified
- Dietary guidelines made easy to follow
- Nutrition labels made understandable
- Vitamins and minerals explained
- Fat-burning foods enumerated
- Meal planning and recipes made doable

Start reaping the benefits of eating healthy and living healthy! You can get started today.

Visit to Order Your Copy Today!
https://www.amazon.com/dp/1519485492

DO YOU WANT TO KNOW HOW YOU CAN LOSE WEIGHT AND BUILD MUSCLE FAST, STARTING RIGHT NOW? THIS BOOK WILL LET YOU IN ON THE SECRET!

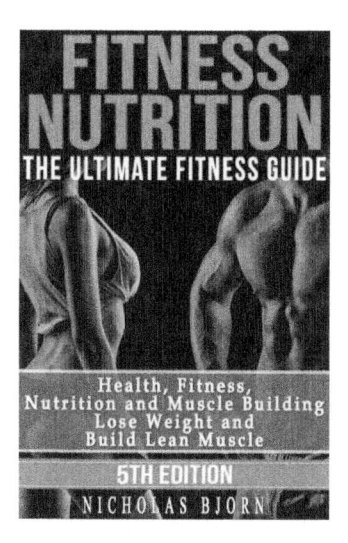

Everyone knows how important it is to maintain a healthy physique. Often, achieving the ideal body requires you to lose weight and build lean muscle. But how do you do that? To become physically fit, you need to have the knowledge necessary to get you on your way and the motivation required to keep you going.

Here's what this book has in store for you:
- Learn how your body uses calories and what role carbohydrates play in your weight
- Discover which foods contain good fats and lean protein that could benefit your body
- Determine what your meal frequency and caloric intake should be
- Know which exercises you should do to get that toned and sculpted look

With the knowledge you will gain from this book, you will be on your way to getting the amazing body that you want!

Visit to Order Your Copy Today!

https://www.amazon.com/dp/1514832968

Printed in Great Britain
by Amazon